SELF-ASSESSMENT OF CURRENT KNOWLEDGE IN PEDIATRICS

By

DAVID S. SMITH, M.D.
Professor of Pediatrics
Temple University
School of Medicine
and
Director of Inpatient Services
St. Christopher's Hospital
for Children
Philadelphia, Pennsylvania

800 MULTIPLE CHOICE QUESTIONS
AND REFERENCED ANSWERS

MEDICAL EXAMINATION PUBLISHING COMPANY, INC.
65-36 Fresh Meadow Lane
Flushing, N.Y. 11365
1972

Library of Congress
Catalog Card Number

78-160718

ISBN 0-87488-256-7

July, 1972

PRINTED IN THE UNITED STATES OF AMERICA

TABLE OF CONTENTS

PREFACE

An attempt has been made to develop questions around current topics in pediatrics which should be of interest to the practitioner, academician and student. The impossible task of reviewing the literature has not been limited to pediatric journals.

It is anticipated and hoped that many of the answers will be questioned by critical readers and that the learning experience provided by this type of exercise will be as satisfying as the one we enjoyed in its preparation.

FOR EACH OF THE FOLLOWING MULTIPLE CHOICE QUESTIONS, SELECT THE ONE APPROPRIATE ANSWER:

ALLERGIC RHINITIS

1. THE ALLERGIC REACTION IS THE RESULT OF THE UNION OF ANTIGEN AND ANTIBODY IN TISSUE CELLS WITH THE RELEASE OF HISTAMINE-LIKE SUBSTANCES. EACH OF THE FOLLOWING IS CORRECT, EXCEPT:
   A. IgE antibodies are not present in nasal secretions
   B. The fungal spore sensitive patient does not have eye irritation unless there is a concomitant pollen sensitivity
   C. Basophils and mast cells are important sources of histamine
   D. Evidence suggests that the dust mite is the main allergic component in house dust
   E. Polymorphonuclear cells are probably concerned in the removal of excess histamine

   Ref. Proc Roy Soc Med 64:447, April 1971

ANTIHUMAN LYMPHOCYTE GLOBULIN, RABBIT

2. THE USE OF RABBIT ANTIHUMAN LYMPHOCYTE GLOBULIN (ALG) IN CADAVER-KIDNEY TRANSPLANTATION HAS BEEN ASSOCIATED WITH ALL OF THE FOLLOWING, EXCEPT:
   A. Rabbit antilymphocyte globulin has caused fewer local and systemic sensitivity reactions than most horse ALG proparations
   B. Acute transplant rejections have been fewer and more easily reversed with the use of rabbit ALG
   C. Rabbit ALG has not been associated with thrombocytopenia which has been a serious complication of horse ALG therapy
   D. The use of ALG permits the administration of relatively low prednisone doses
   E. Rabbit ALG has apparently eliminated "chronic rejection" or progressive loss of transplant function beyond the one-year level in cadaver-kidney transplants

   Ref. New Engl J Med 284:1114, May 20, 1971

ASPERGILLUS AND EOSINOPHILIC INFILTRATIONS

3. A HIGH PROPORTION OF EOSINOPHILIC INFILTRATIONS IN THE LUNGS OF ASTHMATICS WHO HAVE BEEN STUDIED IN GREAT BRITAIN CAN BE RELATED TO ASPERGILLUS FUMIGATUS. THE LATTER IS AN IMPORTANT PATHOGEN OF BIRDS, BOTH WILD AND DOMESTICATED, INFECTING THEIR LUNGS AND AIR-SACS. IN MAN, ASPERGILLUS HAS BEEN ASSOCIATED WITH ALL OF THE FOLLOWING CLINICAL PICTURES, EXCEPT:
   A. The "fungus ball" or aspergilloma, in which the mold colonizes an existing air-containing space in the lung
   B. Aspergillus may grow in devitalized or damaged lung without producing any obvious clinical features
   C. Aspergillus may behave as an opportunistic pathogen in children with Hodgkin's disease or leukemia
   D. In atopic subjects, aspergillus may cause recurrent episodes of localized pulmonary infiltration with blood eosinophilia
   E. Involvement of the pleura and bronchiectasis have not been observed

   Ref. Proc Roy Soc Med 64:381, April 1971

BREAST MILK AND SECRETORY IgA

4. IT HAS BEEN KNOWN FOR MANY YEARS THAT BREAST-FED BABIES HAVE FEWER EPISODES OF DIARRHEAL DISEASE THAN BOTTLE-FED INFANTS. THE ROLE OF SECRETORY IgA IN COLOSTRUM AND BREAST MILK IN THE IMMUNOLOGIC DEFENSE OF THE INFANT'S GUT HAS BEEN EXPLAINED IN ALL OF THE FOLLOWING, EXCEPT:
   A. The amount of secretory IgA decreases rapidly as the transition from colostrum to milk takes place, and negligible amounts remain in milk after lactation is established
   B. Secretory IgA is the major carrier of antibodies in colostrum and breast milk
   C. No secretory IgA has been identified in the serum of an infant who has been breast fed
   D. Colostrum contains live and functional lymphoid cells, as well as effective phagocytic cells
   E. IgA can be seen by immunofluorescent preparations on the luminal surface of the epithelial cells of the infant's gut

   Ref. J Pediat
   76:6, July, 1971

IMMUNOLOGY, X-LINKED DISORDERS

5. MANY OF THE DISORDERS OF RESISTANCE TO INFECTION HAVE AN X-LINKED MODE OF TRANSMISSION. EACH OF THE FOLLOWING FOLLOWS SUCH A PATTERN OF INHERITANCE, EXCEPT:
   A. Bruton's agammaglobulinemia
   B. Wiskott-Aldrich syndrome
   C. Chronic granulomatous disease
   D. Thymic alymphoplasia
   E. Congenital absence of the thymus (DiGeorge Syndrome)

   Ref. Lancet
   2:826, 1969

IMMUNOGLOBULINS

6. THE CONCENTRATIONS OF IMMUNOGLOBULINS VARY FROM ONE INDIVIDUAL TO ANOTHER, AND THERE IS AT PRESENT NO CONCLUSIVE EVIDENCE TO JUSTIFY THRESHOLDS FOR THE DIAGNOSIS OF IMMUNOGLOBULIN DEFICIENCIES. EACH OF THE FOLLOWING STATEMENTS IS CORRECT, EXCEPT:
   A. Normal immunoglobulin levels exclude antibody deficiency
   B. In children with exudative protein-losing enteropathies and in the nephrotic syndrome normal levels of IgM are usually found
   C. IgA is undetectable in the serum of approximately 0.1% of the population
   D. Patients have been found with normal levels of serum IgA and low levels of secretory IgA
   E. X-linked recessive agammaglobulinemia is characterized by very low levels of all five classes of immunoglobulins

   Ref. Pediatrics
   47:931, May, 1971

IMMUNODEFICIENCIES

7. EVIDENCE SUGGESTS THAT STEM CELLS ORIGINATING IN BONE MARROW DIFFERENTIATE TO FORM AT LEAST TWO DISTINCT LYMPHOCYTE POPULATIONS: ONE (T-LYMPHOCYTES) DEPENDENT ON THE PRESENCE OF THE THYMUS, AND THE OTHER (B-LYMPHOCYTES) INDEPENDENT OF THE THYMUS. EACH OF THE FOLLOWING IS ACCEPTED AS CORRECT IN REGARD TO THE ROLE OF THE LYMPHOCYTE, EXCEPT:

A. T- lymphocytes constitute the greater part of the recirculating pool of small lymphocytes
B. B- lymphocytes appear to be more restricted to lymphoid tissue
C. Both populations of lymphocytes contain antigen-sensitive cells, probably with specific antibody on their surface
D. B-lymphocytes can differentiate, proliferate, and mature into plasma cells which synthesize humoral antibody
E. Defects which limit the number and differentiation of the T-lymphocyte lead to deficiencies in the synthesis of immunoglobulins

Ref. Pediatrics
47:927, May, 1971

ISOPROTERENOL AND ASTHMA

8. THE USE OF INTRAVENOUS ISOPROTERENOL IN STATUS ASTHMATICUS MAY LESSEN THE NEED FOR INTUBATION AND MECHANICAL VENTILATION. IN A GROUP OF CHILDREN TREATED WITH THIS TECHNIQUE ALL OF THE FOLLOWING HAVE BEEN SUGGESTED, EXCEPT:

A. Isoproterenol is a potent bronchodilator
B. ECG monitoring is suggested because of the possibility of ventricular arrhythmias
C. Enzyme studies have suggested the possibility of heart-muscle damage in some children
D. Frequent arterial blood gas determinations are mandatory
E. Intubation and mechanical ventilation have led to infection, pneumothorax and tracheal stenosis

Ref. Medical World News
12:33, November 12, 1971

JOB'S SYNDROME

9. JOB'S SYNDROME IS AN IMMUNOLOGIC DISEASE WHICH ORIGINALLY WAS DESCRIBED IN FAIR-SKINNED, RED-HEADED FEMALES. EACH OF THE FOLLOWING IS CORRECT, EXCEPT:

A. The disease is characterized by recurrent cold, non-tender abscesses
B. Eosinophilia has been a striking characteristic of biopsy material from abscess sites
C. Biopsies of skin and abscesses have demonstrated histiocytes loaded with pigmented lipid as has been characteristic of chronic granulomatous disease
D. The nature of the defect in Job's syndrome has not been recognized
E. Leukocytes from girls with Job's syndrome have shown normal reduction of nitro blue tetrazolium following phagocytosis

Ref. J Pediatr
75:235, August, 1969
Immunology Section, APS/SPR
Atlantic City, April 30, 1971

LYMPHOCYTES

10. FAILURE TO DEVELOP AN EFFECTIVE THYMIC-DEPENDENT LYMPHOCYTE SYSTEM (T-CELL) LEADS TO DEFECTS IN CELL-MEDIATED IMMUNITY. OTHER CHARACTERISTICS OF THE T-CELL INCLUDE ALL OF THE FOLLOWING, EXCEPT:
    A. T-cells can be nonspecifically stimulated in culture by mitogens, such as phytohemagglutinin
    B. T-cells have a short life span
    C. They may be "killer" cells which are cytotoxic for graft target cells
    D. They may cooperate during the immune response to certain ("thymus-dependent") antigens by stimulating the B-lymphocyte (independent of the thymus) to produce antibody
    E. They release a number of soluble factors which are chemotactic for mononuclear cells and inhibit the migration of macrophages

    Ref. Pediatrics
    47:928, May, 1971

ANTIBODIES, ASSESSMENT OF

11. HUMORAL IMMUNITY FUNCTION MAY BE STUDIED BY TESTS FOR EXISTING ANTIBODIES TO ANTIGENS TO WHICH THE POPULATION IS COMMONLY EXPOSED, OR BY TESTS FOR ANTIBODY FORMATION AFTER CERTAIN ACTIVE IMMUNIZATIONS. ALL OF THE FOLLOWING ARE RECOMMENDED IN THE ASSESSMENT OF HUMORAL IMMUNITY, EXCEPT:
    A. "Natural" antibodies such as A and B isohemagglutins
    B. Active immunization with diphtheria, tetanus and pertussis (DPT)
    C. Inactivated polio vaccine
    D. Immunization with polysaccharides derived from pneumococci, H. influenzae and N. meningitides antigens
    E. BCG

    Ref. Pediatrics
    47:932, May 1971

CELL-MEDIATED IMMUNITY, ASSESSMENT OF

12. DELAYED-TYPE SKIN REACTIONS ARE COMMONLY EMPLOYED FOR ASSESSING CELL-MEDIATED IMMUNITY. ALL OF THE FOLLOWING ANTIGENS ARE RECOMMENDED FOR THIS EVALUATION, EXCEPT:
    A. Purified protein derivative (tuberculin)
    B. Candida (1.10 dilution for infants with 1:1,000 for older children and adults)
    C. Trichophytin, as for candida
    D. Mumps skin-testing antigen
    E. Schick test

    Ref. Pediatrics
    47:933, May 1971

IMMUNODEFICIENCIES AND LYMPH NODES

13. EXAMINATION OF LYMPHOID TISSUE AND BONE MARROW ARE USEFUL TOOLS IN THE DIAGNOSIS OF IMMUNE DEFICIENCY STATES. EACH OF THE FOLLOWING IS CORRECT, EXCEPT:
    A. Tonsil and adenoid tissue may be absent in certain immunodeficiencies
    B. No diagnosis of immunodeficiency is tenable without a lymph node biopsy
    C. In young infants enumeration of bone marrow lymphoid cells may not be helpful in the diagnosis of immunodeficiencies
    D. Deficiencies of lymphocytes in the deep cortical regions of lymph nodes indicate defects of the T-cell system (thymic dependent)
    E. Plasma cells and germinal centers are absent in lymph nodes in most complete isolated B-cell deficiencies (not thymus dependent)

    Ref. Pediatrics
    47:936, May, 1971

IMMUNODEFICIENCIES - MISCELLANEOUS

14. ADDITIONAL HISTOPATHOLOGIC OR LABORATORY EXAMINATIONS MAY LEAD TO CLUES IN THE DIAGNOSIS OF IMMUNODEFICIENCIES. EACH OF THE FOLLOWING STATEMENTS IS CORRECT, EXCEPT:
A. Absence of plasma cells from the lamina propria in a rectal biopsy reflects deficiency of the local IgA immunoglobulin system
B. In severe combined immunodeficiency the blood lymphocyte count is always markedly depressed
C. Low serum IgM concentration in the second and subsequent weeks of life may help in the diagnosis of immunodeficiency
D. Immunity function tests should be performed in all cases of neonatal tetany
E. Chimerism (two genetically different cell lines) due to intrauterine transfer of maternal cells into the fetus has been demonstrated in immunoincompetent infants

Ref. Pediatrics 47:936, May, 1971

MITES, HOUSE DUST ALLERGY

15. THE ANTIGENIC FACTOR IN HOUSE DUST HAS BEEN THE SUBJECT OF MANY YEARS OF INVESTIGATION. AN ORIGINAL REPORT BY VAN LEEUWEN IN 1922 SUGGESTING MITES AS A POSSIBLE ALLERGEN IN HOUSE DUST HAS BEEN THE OBJECT OF RENEWED INTEREST IN RECENT LITERATURE. EACH OF THE FOLLOWING IS CORRECT, EXCEPT:
A. Mite counts are usually higher in articles of furniture which are used by humans both day and night, such as day beds
B. Dermatophagoides pteronyssinus, or the common house mite, is usually present in mattresses or furniture stuffed with cotton fiber
C. Most patients who show positive skin reactions to house dust extract also show positive reactions to the extract of mites but not vice-versa
D. Extracts of dust where no mites are found are usually inert on the skin of dust sensitive individuals
E. The excretions of mites contain the same or similar skin reacting antigens as the whole organism

Ref. Ann Allerg 27:93, March, 1969

PNEUMOCOCCAL SEPSIS

16. DISSEMINATED INTRAVASCULAR COAGULATION OCCURRING AS THE RESULT OF PNEUMOCOCCAL SEPSIS APPEARS TO BE A SIGNIFICANT RISK IN CHILDREN WITH:
A. Hypergammaglobulinemia
B. Chronic granulomatous disease
C. Chediak-Higashi syndrome
D. DiGeorge syndrome
E. Hyposplenism or postsplenectomy

Ref. Ann Intern Med 72:389, March 1970

FOR EACH OF THE FOLLOWING QUESTIONS, SELECT THE <u>ONE</u> APPROPRIATE ANSWER BY USING THE KEY OUTLINED BELOW:

1. If A, B and C are correct
2. If A and C are correct
3. If B and D are correct
4. If all are correct
5. If all are incorrect

<u>CHRONIC GRANULOMATOUS DISEASE</u>

17. SIGNS AND SYMPTOMS WHICH ARE FOUND IN OVER HALF OF CHILDREN WITH CHRONIC GRANULOMATOUS DISEASE INCLUDE:
A. Marked lymphadenopathy
B. Pneumonitis
C. Hepatomegaly
D. Arthritis
E. Perianal abscess

Ref. Pediatrics
48:730, November, 1971

18. THE CRITICAL LESION OF THE CHRONIC GRANULOMATOUS DISEASE PHAGOCYTE IS ITS INABILITY TO GENERATE HYDROGEN PEROXIDE, WHICH ALLOWS INGESTED BACTERIA TO SURVIVE. WHICH OF THE FOLLOWING BACTERIA FORM THEIR OWN PEROXIDE AND ALLOW KILLING BY THE CGD PHAGOCYTE?:
A. Staphylococci
B. Streptococci
C. Candida albicans
D. Pneumococci
E. Gram-negative enterics

Ref. Pediatrics
48:730, November, 1971

19. THE SUCCESSFUL TREATMENT OF CHRONIC GRANULOMATOUS DISEASE HAS BEEN ACCOMPLISHED WITH WHICH OF THE FOLLOWING?:
A. Methylene blue to increase pentose shunt activity
B. Vitamin A to promote release of lysosomal enzymes
C. Corticosteroids
D. Gamma globulin
E. Leukocyte transfusions

Ref. Pediatrics
48:730, November, 1971

<u>FIFTH COMPONENT OF COMPLEMENT</u>

20. A SECOND FAMILY WITH A DEFICIENCY OF PHAGOCYTOSIS ENHANCEMENT (OPSONIZATION) RELATED TO A DYSFUNCTION OF THE FIFTH COMPONENT OF COMPLEMENT HAS BEEN DESCRIBED. THE CLINICAL SPECTRUM INCLUDES WHICH OF THE FOLLOWING?:
A. Recurrent local and systemic infections, usually of gram-negative etiology
B. Chronic seborrheic dermatitis
C. Intractable, severe diarrhea
D. Marked wasting
E. Improvement with fresh plasma transfusions

Ref. Pediatrics
49:225, 1972

HYPERIMMUNOGLOBINEMIA E

21. CONDITIONS WHICH HAVE BEEN ASSOCIATED WITH ELEVATED SERUM CONCENTRATIONS OF IgE HAVE INCLUDED WHICH OF THE FOLLOWING?:
A. Wiskott-Aldrich syndrome
B. Atopic diseases
C. Parasitic infestations
D. Pulmonary hemosiderosis
E. Multiple myeloma

Ref. Pediatrics
49:59, January, 1972

22. A NEW SYNDROME CHARACTERIZED BY EXTREME HYPERIMMUNOGLOBULINEMIA E AND UNDUE SUSCEPTIBILITY TO INFECTION HAS BEEN ASSOCIATED WITH WHICH OF THE FOLLOWING?:
A. Eosinophilia
B. Recurrent bacterial and fungal infection
C. Impaired cell-mediated immunity
D. Subnormal antibody formation
E. Chronic dermatitis

Ref. Pediatrics
49:59, January, 1972

IgA DEFICIENCY, ABNORMALITIES ASSOCIATED WITH

23. WHICH OF THE FOLLOWING HAVE BEEN ASSOCIATED WITH SELECTIVE IgA DEFICIENCY?:
A. Chromosome 18 abnormalities
B. Sprue-like syndromes
C. Autoimmune disorders
D. Allergy
E. Healthy children

Ref. Pediatrics
49:71, January, 1972

IgA, FAMILIAL SELECTIVE DEFICIENCY

24. FAMILIES IN WHOM SELECTIVE IgA DEFICIENCY HAS BEEN DISCOVERED HAVE DEMONSTRATED WHICH OF THE FOLLOWING?:
A. Low isohemagglutinins
B. Autosomal pattern of inheritance in some
C. Abnormal response to diphtheria toxin
D. Increased autoantibody production
E. Abnormal peripheral lymphocyte response to phytohemagglutinin

Ref. Pediatrics
49:71, January, 1972

IgA DEFICIENCY AND OTHER IMMUNOLOGIC ABNORMALITIES

25. SELECTIVE IgA DEFICIENCY HAS HAD AN ASSOCIATION WITH WHICH OF THE FOLLOWING IMMUNOLOGIC ABNORMALITIES?:
A. Rubella syndrome
B. Thymic hypoplasia
C. Ataxia-telangiectasia
D. Wiscott-Aldrich
E. Aleutian mink disease

Ref. Pediatrics
49:71, January, 1972

IMMUNE SUPPRESSION

26. SUPPRESSION OF DELAYED HYPERSENSITIVITY REACTIONS IN THE IMMUNE RESPONSE MAY BE QUICKLY ACCOMPLISHED BY WHICH OF THE FOLLOWING?:
A. Corticosteroids
B. Actinomycin
C. Antilymphocyte globulin
D. Thymectomy
E. Splenectomy

Ref. J Med Genet
8:321, September, 1971

IgM, ELEVATED IN NEWBORN INFANTS

27. SCREENING CORD SERUM IgM FOR EVIDENCE OF INTRAUTERINE INFECTIONS HAS LED TO WHICH OF THE FOLLOWING FINDINGS:
A. Infants with obvious congenital infections often have elevated levels of IgM
B. A disproportionate number of false-positives
C. Many false-negatives
D. An increase in structural defects in infants with elevated IgM over controls
E. An increased incidence of major and minor neuromotor abnormalities in infants with elevated IgM

Ref. J Pediatr
78:1020, 1971

THYROTOXICOSIS, NEONATAL AND INFANTILE

28. WHICH OF THE FOLLOWING STATEMENTS ARE CORRECT CONCERNING GRAVE'S DISEASE IN THE VERY YOUNG?:
A. Long-acting thyroid stimulator (LATS) is always identified in patients with hyperthyroidism
B. The degree of thyrotoxicosis correlates with the concentration of LATS
C. Neonatal hyperthyroidism does not persist after the disappearance of LATS
D. Evidence suggests that the underlying defect in thyrotoxicosis is not genetically determined
E. Neonatal thyrotoxicosis is a self-limited pathophysiologic state

Ref. Calif Med
113:50, 1970

TRANSPLANTATION, BONE MARROW

29. BONE-MARROW TRANSPLANTATION IN THE LYMPHOPENIC IMMUNOLOGIC DEFICIENCY SYNDROMES HAS BEEN ASSOCIATED WITH WHICH OF THE FOLLOWING OBSERVATIONS?:
A. Immunoglobulin levels may rise in a sequential order following transplantation corresponding to their ontogenetic development
B. Successful transplantation has been associated with red-cell development
C. Immunologic reconstitution has been successful in lymphopenic immunologic deficiency states which have included the Swiss type and the Wiscott-Aldrich syndrome
D. Despite successful transplantation lymph nodes do not become palpable in the weeks which follow
E. The use of bone-marrow cells from an HL-A identical sibling and a negative mixed lymphocyte culture between the donor and the recipient has eliminated the graft-vs.-host reaction

Ref. New Eng J Med
285:1399, December 16, 1971

ANEMIA

ANEMIA IN CHILDREN MAY BE DUE TO THE FOLLOWING CAUSES OF EXCESSIVE DESTRUCTION OF RED BLOOD CELLS. MATCH THE CAUSE WITH THE CLINICAL DIAGNOSIS:

A. Formation of abnormal red cells
B. Formation of red cells "hypersusceptible" to hemolysis
C. Presence of "extracorpuscular" factors

30. ___ Hypersplenism
31. ___ Thalassemia
32. ___ Pyruvate kinase deficiency
33. ___ Cold agglutinins
34. ___ Glucose-6-phosphate dehydrogenase deficiency
35. ___ Paroxysmal nocturnal hemoglobinuria
36. ___ Hemolytic uremic syndrome
37. ___ Hereditary spherocytosis
38. ___ Anemia of collagen disease
39. ___ Autoimmune hemolytic anemia

Ref. Pediat Clin N Amer 18:16, February, 1971

ANEMIA, LABORATORY TESTS

ANEMIA IS A SYMPTOM WHICH MUST HAVE A DEFINITION FOR PROPER MANAGEMENT. IN THE FOLLOWING LIST OF CONFIRMATORY TESTS WHICH ARE HELPFUL IN THE DIAGNOSIS OF ANEMIA, MATCH THE ONE STATEMENT IN THE RIGHT HAND COLUMN WHICH BEST APPLIES TO THE STATEMENT IN THE LEFT HAND COLUMN:

40. ___ Electronic red cell count
41. ___ Heinz bodies
42. ___ Acid hemolysis
43. ___ Hemoglobin A_2 percentage
44. ___ Coombs' test (direct)
45. ___ Hemoglobin F slide test
46. ___ Folic acid level
47. ___ Osmotic fragility
48. ___ Red cell enzyme assay
49. ___ Presence of methalbuminemia

A. Hereditary spherocytosis
B. Glucose-6-phosphate dehydrogenase deficiency
C. Red cell size, red cell indices
D. Paroxysmal nocturnal hemoglobinuria
E. Thalassemia
F. Drug induced hemolysis
G. Recent intravascular hemolysis
H. Fetal-maternal bleeding
I. Autoimmune hemolytic anemia
J. Absorption defect

Ref. Pediat Clin N Amer 18:16, February, 1971

HEMOLYTIC ANEMIAS

ALTHOUGH THE CAUSE FOR HEMOLYSIS OF RED BLOOD CELLS IS INCOMPLETELY UNDERSTOOD IN MANY DISORDERS, MATCH THE MOST LIKELY CAUSE FOR PREMATURE DESTRUCTION OF CIRCULATING ERYTHROCYTES WITH THE REPRESENTATIVE EXAMPLE:

A. Abnormalities of hemoglobin influencing the flow properties of the red cells
B. Exposure of red cells to inordinate physical trauma in the circulation
C. Abnormalities associated with the red cell membrane

50. ___ Hemoglobin S
51. ___ Immunohemolytic anemias
52. ___ Hereditary spherocytosis
53. ___ March hemoglobinuria
54. ___ Disseminated intravascular coagulation
55. ___ Oxidant drugs (G-6-PD deficiency)

Ref. New Eng J Med 285:1514, December 30, 1971

LEUKEMIA

THE IDENTIFICATION OF THE CELL LINE INVOLVED IN CHILDHOOD LEUKEMIA IS IMPORTANT IN OUTLINING THERAPY AND IN DETERMINING PROGNOSIS. ALTHOUGH NONE OF THE NEWER TECHNICS OF STAINING, CHROMOSOME ANALYSIS OR CELL CULTURE ARE ABSOLUTE IN DIFFERENTIATING THE LEUKEMIC CELL. MATCH THE TYPE WITH THE APPROPRIATE LABORATORY AND CLINICAL SIGN:

A. Acute lymphocytic leukemia
B. Acute or chronic myelogenous leukemia
C. Both
D. Neither

56. ___ Bone pain
57. ___ Central nervous system involvement
58. ___ Sudan Black and peroxidase staining
59. ___ Chromosome analysis
60. ___ Increased proportion of fetal hemoglobin
61. ___ Periodic acid-Shiff staining

Ref. Clin Pediat
10:571, October, 1971

MEGALOBLASTIC ANEMIAS

MATCH THE THREE TYPES OF VITAMIN B_{12} RESPONSIVE MEGALOBLASTIC ANEMIAS OF INFANCY WITH THE EXPECTED CLINICAL AND LABORATORY FINDINGS:

A. Deficiency of vitamin B_{12} transport protein (transcolbalamin II)
B. Defective intestinal absorption of B_{12}
C. Lack of intrinsic-factor activity in gastric juice

62. ___ Low serum vitamin B_{12}, normal gastric mucosa, free hydrochloric acid present, strong familial tendency
63. ___ Early onset, strong familial occurence, generalized and persistent proteinuria, low serum vitamin B_{12}, may have generalized malabsorption
64. ___ Normal levels of vitamin B_{12}, response to massive doses of B_{12} per week, absence of any signs of deficiency at birth autosomal recessive disease

Ref. New Eng J Med
285:1163, November 18, 1971

FOR EACH OF THE FOLLOWING MULTIPLE CHOICE QUESTIONS, SELECT THE ONE APPROPRIATE ANSWER:

ASPIRIN AND BLEEDING

65. ASPIRIN IS ABSOLUTELY CONTRAINDICATED IN CHILDREN WITH BLEEDING DISORDERS AND IN THOSE WHO ARE UNDERGOING SURGICAL PROCEDURES BECAUSE OF ITS EFFECT ON "PLATELET AGGREGATION." ALL OF THE FOLLOWING STATEMENTS ARE CORRECT, EXCEPT:

A. Aspirin inhibits the release of endogenous adenosine diphosphate, thus preventing the aggregation of platelets
B. Altered platelet function in newborn infants has not been related to the maternal ingestion of aspirin
C. Platelet abnormalities caused by aspirin may persist for 4 to 7 days
D. Aspirin induced bleeding has been linked to post-tonsillectomy hemorrhage
E. As little as 5 grains of aspirin can produce platelet abnormalities

Ref. Infectious Diseases
1:3, August, 1971

DISSEMINATED INTRAVASCULAR COAGULATION

66. DISSEMINATED INTRAVASCULAR COAGULATION HAS BEEN ASSOCIATED WITH A WIDE SPECTRUM OF CLINICAL PROBLEMS. THE DIAGNOSIS IS SUPPORTED BY FINDING ALL OF THE FOLLOWING LABORATORY ABNORMALITIES, EXCEPT:
A. Absence of fibrin split products in the serum
B. Thrombocytopenia
C. Prolonged thrombin time
D. Anemia with red cell fragmentation
E. Abnormal prothrombin and partial thromboplastin times

Ref. Pediatric News
5:1, June, 1971

67. MOST AUTHORITIES AGREE THAT BETTER CRITERIA ARE NEEDED FOR THE DIAGNOSIS OF DISSEMINATED INTRAVASCULAR COAGULATION. ALL OF THE FOLLOWING ARE ACCEPTED AS CORRECT, EXCEPT:
A. Hypotension and shock are usually absent in DIC associated with viral diseases
B. The value of heparin therapy in the treatment of DIC has not been established
C. DIC is rarely observed in newborns
D. DIC associated with bacterial sepsis is associated frequently with hypotension and shock
E. DIC has been associated with such unrelated clinical problems as the giant cavernous hemangioma and the battered child syndrome with massive skull fracture

Ref. Pediatric News
5:30, June, 1971

DISSEMINATED INTRAVASCULAR COAGULATION IN THE NEWBORN

68. THE THERAPY OF DISSEMINATED INTRAVASCULAR COAGULATION IN THE NEWBORN HAS BEEN ASSOCIATED WITH ALL OF THE FOLLOWING, EXCEPT:
A. The fibrinolytic phase of DIC may be prolonged by the slow clearance of heparin
B. The generalized Shwartzman reaction in the newborn may be enhanced by recent and prolonged exposure to estrogens
C. The hypoxia accompanying severe respiratory distress may initiate damage to tissue which is rich in clotting factors
D. The clotting defects of DIC may be corrected by exchange transfusion
E. The correction of the consumptive coagulopathy by transfusion depends upon the use of fresh whole citrated blood

Ref. J Pediatr
78:415, March, 1971

ERYTHROPOIETIN

69. SEVERAL OBJECTIONS EXIST TO MAKING THE KIDNEY THE SOLE SITE FOR THE PRODUCTION AND RELEASE OF ERYTHROPOIETIN. EACH OF THE FOLLOWING HAS BEEN OBSERVED IN THE SEARCH FOR ERYTHROPOIETIN, EXCEPT:
A. It has not been possible to isolate appreciable amounts of erythropoietin from kidney homogenate
B. Bilateral carotid-body removal in cats results in a rapid drop in hematocrit values
C. Injections of carotid-body extract or blood from carotid-body efferent vessels causes pronounced increases in reticulocyte counts and in iron utilization
D. Severe hypoxia in the anephric human may cause the release of small amounts of erythropoietin
E. The large renal blood supply tends to make the kidney exquisitely sensitive to small changes in hemoglobin thus supporting the concept of the kidney as an oxygen-sensing apparatus controlling the release of erythropoietin

Ref. New Eng J Med 284:849, April 15, 1971

HEMOLYSIS OF RED CELLS

70. THE MECHANISMS OF HEMOLYSIS OF RED BLOOD CELLS INVOLVE ALL OF THE FOLLOWING, EXCEPT:
A. The most critical measure of plasticity of RBC's is their ability to traverse the spleen filter
B. Vitamin E deficiency contributes to hemolysis in premature infants
C. Hemolysis in uremia is usually mild
D. The major cause of anemia in chronic renal failure is decreased red-cell production
E. Hemolytic anemia occurs with chronic fat malabsorption in older children

Ref. New Eng J Med 285:1514, December 30, 1971

HEMOLYTIC-UREMIC SYNDROME

71. WHICH OF THE FOLLOWING HAS NOT BEEN DEMONSTRATED AS PART OF THE DISSEMINATED INTRAVASCULAR COAGULATION WHICH ACCOMPANIES THE HEMOLYTIC-UREMIC SYNDROME ?:
A. Circulating endotoxin
B. Intracapillary thrombi
C. Renal cortical necrosis
D. Microangiopathic hemolytic anemia
E. Shortened Cr_{51} platelet survival

Ref. J Pediatr 80:1, January, 1972

HEMORRHAGIC DISEASE OF THE NEWBORN

72. EACH OF THE FOLLOWING STATEMENTS IN REGARD TO HEMORRHAGIC DISEASE OF THE NEWBORN IS CORRECT, EXCEPT:
A. Vitamin K activity of human breast milk is equal to that of cow's milk
B. A rapid response of prothrombin activity follows the first feeding of cow's milk within hours
C. Many infants receiving human milk have normal prothrombin values
D. Parenterally administered vitamin K promptly corrects a prolonged prothrombin time
E. Total starvation combined with antibiotic therapy results in a decrease in vitamin K dependent coagulation factors

Ref. Amer J Dis Child 121:271, April, 1971

HOWELL-JOLLY BODIES

73. HOWELL-JOLLY BODIES ARE NUCLEAR REMNANTS PRESENT IN ERYTHROCYTES. THE NUCLEAR ORIGIN IS SUGGESTED BY THEIR AFFINITY FOR STAINS SUCH AS METHYL GREEN WHICH IS SPECIFIC FOR CHROMATIN. EACH OF THE FOLLOWING IS ASSOCIATED WITH HOWELL-JOLLY BODIES, EXCEPT:

A. Malaria
B. Thalassemia
C. Leukemia
D. Postsplenectomy
E. Congenital absence of the spleen

Ref. Diagnostica
Number 20, May, 1971, p.24

IRON-DEFICIENCY ANEMIA AT BIRTH

74. A NEWBORN INFANT, IN NO ACUTE DISTRESS, IS BORN TO AN O Rh POSITIVE MOTHER WITH A HEMOGLOBIN OF 4.5gms. THE HEMATOCRIT IS 11 PER CENT, AND THE RETICULOCYTE COUNT 31 PER CENT. THE INFANT'S PERIPHERAL BLOOD SMEAR CONTAINS HYPOCHROMIC, MICROCYTIC ERYTHROCYTES WITH POIKIOLOCYTOSIS, ANISOCYTOSIS, TEARDROP CELLS, MARKED POLYCHROMATOPHILIA AND OCCASIONAL BASOPHILIC STIPPLING. THERE IS NO ORGANOMEGALY. THE MOST USEFUL LABORATORY TEST IN MAKING A DIAGNOSIS WOULD BE:

A. Hemoglobin F concentration in the mother (normal adult level less than 2 percent)
B. A direct Coomb's test on the infant
C. Red blood cell saline fragility studies on the infant
D. Major blood grouping and typing of maternal and infant red blood cells
E. A bone marrow examination on the infant

Ref. Clin Pediat
10:223, April, 1971

LAZY LEUKOCYTE SYNDROME

75. THE "LAZY LEUKOCYTE SYNDROME," A NEW DISORDER OF NEUTROPHIL FUNCTION HAS BEEN ADDED TO CHRONIC GRANULOMATOUS DESEASE AS A CAUSE OF RECURRENT INFECTIONS RELATED TO AN INTRINSIC DEFICIENCY OF THE NEUTROPHIL. EACH OF THE FOLLOWING IS TRUE IN REGARD TO THIS SYNDROME, EXCEPT:

A. The primary abnormality of leukocyte function appears to be a defect in chemotaxis
B. Neutrophils from peripheral blood and bone marrow have normal phagocytic activity
C. Neutrophils from peripheral blood and bone marrow have normal bactericidal activity
D. Severe peripheral neutropenia is characteristic
E. An appreciable increase in the total white blood cell count or in the absolute number of polymorphonuclear leukocytes follows adrenalin or piromen stimulation

Ref. Lancet
1:665, April 3, 1971

LEUKEMIA AND METABOLIC ALKALOSIS

76. A CHILD WHO IS UNDER TREATMENT FOR ACUTE LYMPHOCYTIC LEUKEMIA, WHO DEVELOPS MUSCLE WEAKNESS, CONSTIPATION, POLYDIPSIA, HYPOSTHENURIA, A DECREASED QT INTERVAL AND T AND P WAVE FLATTENING OR INVERSION, AND A METABOLIC ALKALOSIS SHOULD BE SUSPECTED OF:

A. Hyperkalemia
B. Hypernatremia
C. Hypercalcemia
D. Hyponatremia
E. Hypochloremia

Ref. J. Pediatr
78:861, May, 1971

LEUKEMIA AND TOTAL THERAPY

77. "TOTAL THERAPY" IN ACUTE LYMPHOCYTIC LEUKEMIA HAS ATTAINED A SIGNIFICANT FIVE-YEAR CURE RATE OF A FATAL DESEASE. EACH OF THE FOLLOWING IS CORRECT IN REGARD TO THE NEWER ASPECTS OF TREATMENT, EXCEPT:

A. It is possible in most children with acute lymphocytic leukemia to induce early remission with vincristine and prednisone
B. Hepatic fibrosis can be caused by chemotherapy with methotrexate or mercaptopurine
C. There has been an unexplained predominance in males in those children with a five-year cure rate
D. After the initial induction of a remission intensive therapy is instituted with antimetabolites
E. Irradiation is now unnecessary to inhibit or destroy residual leukemic cells in the central nervous system and is not part of the "total therapy" of childhood lymphocytic leukemia

Ref. JAMA
216:648, April 26, 1971

RH_O (D) IMMUNE GLOBULIN (HUMAN)

78. ISOIMMUNIZATION TO THE RH FACTOR MAY BE PREVENTED BY PASSIVE IMMUNIZATION WITH RH_O (D) IMMUNE GLOBULIN (HUMAN). ALL OF THE FOLLOWING ARE CORRECT IN REGARD TO RH_O(D) IMMUNE GLOBULIN (HUMAN), EXCEPT:

A. There are 72 hours available postpartum or following abortion for effective administration
B. It should not be administered to an Rh (D) positive or D^u individual
C. It may be given to the infant in cases of mild sensitization
D. It should not be given to a mother who has been previously sensitized to Rh (D)
E. It should not be given to an individual who has recently received an Rh (D) positive blood transfusion

Ref. Am Col Obstet Gynecol
13, June, 1970

METHEMOGLOBINEMIA AND WELL WATER

79. DRINKING WATER CONTAINING HIGH LEVELS OF NITRATES CONTINUES TO PRESENT THE HAZARD OF METHEMOGLOBINEMIA FROM NUMEROUS RURAL WELLS IN THE UNITED STATES. EACH OF THE FOLLOWING IS CORRECT, EXCEPT:
A. A clear relationship exists between bacterial contamination of wells and high nitrate content
B. Cyanosis in infants occurs when the level of methemoglobin reaches 10 per cent
C. Symptoms related to hypoxia occur when the levels of methemoglobin exceed 20 per cent
D. Infants may be protected from nitrates by the addition of lactic acid to a milk formula
E. Infants seem to be more susceptible than adults to developing methemoglobinemia from the ingestion of water containing excessive nitrates

Ref. JAMA
216:1642, June 7, 1971

PRIAPISM AND SICKLE CELL ANEMIA

80. PRIAPISM IS A PAINFUL AND DIFFICULT COMPLICATION OF SICKLE CELL DISEASE AND REPRESENTS A MECHANICAL OBSTRUCTION OF THE CORPUS CAVERNOSUM WITH SICKLED ERYTHROCYTES. THE MOST SUCCESSFUL METHOD OF TREATMENT APPEARS TO BE:
A. Transfusion of packed erythrocytes
B. Caudal anesthesia
C. Aspiration of the corpus cavernosum and irrigation with heparin
D. Fibrinolytic agents
E. Systemic anticoagulants

Ref. Clin Pediatr
10:418, July, 1971

Rh SENSITIZATION AND ABORTION

81. IT IS CRUCIAL TO IDENTIFY THE RISK OF Rh SENSITIZATION IN INDUCED ABORTIONS TO DETERMINE IF A PROGRAM OF PROPHYLAXIS WITH Rh-IMMUNE GLOBULIN IS NECESSARY. THE ROLE OF INDUCED ABORTION IN RHESUS IMMUNIZATION HAS SHOWN ALL OF THE FOLLOWING, EXCEPT:
A. The Rh antigen is present on the fetal red blood cell as early as the 38th day of gestation
B. The frequency of transplacental hemorrhage in induced abortions decreases with gestation
C. Transplacental hemorrhage occurs in about one-fifth of women whose pregnancy is terminated by hypertonic saline
D. Transplacental hemorrhage occurs in about one in twenty women whose pregnancy is terminated by suction curettage
E. The absence of detectable fetal cells in the maternal circulation does not give assurance that the mother will not become immunized

Ref. Lancet
1:815, April 24, 1971

PURPURA, HENOCH-SCHONLEIN

82. HENOCH-SCHONLEIN PURPURA IS MOST COMMONLY A DISEASE OF CHILDREN. THERE ARE FEW PROBLEMS IN THE DIAGNOSIS OF A TYPICAL CASE WITH ITS CHARACTERISTIC RASH, ARTHRALGIA, ABDOMINAL PAIN AND NEPHRITIS. IN HENOCH-SCHONLEIN PURPURA ALL OF THE FOLLOWING ARE CORRECT EXCEPT:

A. The cutaneous vasculitis syndromes have been classified according to the size of the vessels affected. With large vessel involvement there is an increased association of serious systemic lesions
B. There is immunofluorescent evidence that antigen-antibody complexes are sometimes present in the skin and kidney in Henoch-Schonlein purpura
C. Streptococcal infections are held responsible for the majority of cases
D. There is inadequate evidence that steroids and other immunosuppressant drugs drastically alter the natural course of the disease
E. The majority of children with renal involvement clear completely within a month and are left with no detectable kidney damage

Ref. Br Med J
20:416, February, 1971

SICKLE CELL DISEASE

83. PAINFUL VASO-OCCLUSIVE CRISES IN SICKLE CELL DISEASE INCLUDE ALL OF THE FOLLOWING, EXCEPT:

A. The hand-foot syndrome leaves no permanent sequelae in the metacarpals and metatarsals
B. Levels of serum bilirubin in excess of 25 mg/100 ml are diagnostic of biliary obstruction by a stone in the common duct
C. Areas of bone infarction and periostitis may be invisible by X-ray for the first week
D. Although signs of peritoneal irritation are sometimes present in abdominal crises, audible peristalsis may help to differentiate this type of involvement from appendicitis and peritonitis
E. Angiographic studies in central nervous system infarcts should be avoided in the early stages because of the high tonicity of contrast media

Ref. Pediatrics
48:632, October, 1971

UREA AND SICKLE CRISES

84. THE USE OF UREA IN THE TREATMENT OF SICKLE CRISIS HAS RECEIVED FAVORABLE COMMENT IN THE LAY PRESS, FOR THE PRESENT, THE USE OF INTRAVENOUS UREA IN THIS COMMON PROBLEM SHOULD BE ATTEMPTED WITH CAUTION, AND ITS RESULTS VIEWED WITH A HEALTHY SKEPTICISM. EACH OF THE FOLLOWING IS CORRECT, EXCEPT:

A. Sickling is aggravated by hypertonicity of body fluids
B. Dehydration may encourage sickling
C. Urea produces necrosis of tissue if extravasation occurs
D. Headache has been a side effect of the use of intravenous urea
E. The potential hazard of intravenous urea as a diuretic has not been a problem in its use in sickle crisis

Ref. N Engl J Med
284:913, April 22, 1971

VON WILLEBRAND'S DISEASE

85. IN 1926 VON WILLEBRAND DESCRIBED A FAMILIAL HEMORRHAGIC DISORDER WHICH DIFFERED FROM CLASSIC HEMOPHILIA BY HAVING A PROLONGED BLEEDING TIME AND BY ITS AUTOSOMAL PATTERN OF INHERITANCE. VON WILLEBRAND'S DISEASE IS CHARACTERIZED BY ALL OF THE FOLLOWING, EXCEPT:
A. A deficiency of factor VIII (antihemophilic globulin) in many cases
B. A deficiency of P.A.P.F. (platelet adhesiveness plasma factor)
C. Absence of a primary platelet defect
D. Abnormal platelet function tests
E. Correcting of the bleeding defect with cryoprecipitate
Ref. Lancet
1:No. 7696, February 27, 1971

FOR EACH OF THE FOLLOWING QUESTIONS, SELECT THE ONE APPROPRIATE ANSWER BY USING THE KEY OUTLINED BELOW:
1. If A, B and C are correct
2. If A and C are correct
3. If B and D are correct
4. If all are correct
5. If all are incorrect

BILIRUBIN AND BRAIN DAMAGE

86. WHICH OF THE FOLLOWING ENHANCE THE SUSCEPTIBILITY OF NEWBORN INFANTS TO THE TOXICITY OF BILIRUBIN?:
A. Hypoxia
B. Prematurity
C. Acidosis
D. Hypoglycemia
E. Hypoalbuminemia
Ref. Pediatrics
47:689, 1971

BLOOD TRANSFUSIONS

87. 2, 3-DIPHOSPHOGLYCERATE IS THE PRIMARY FACTOR IN DETERMINING THE POSITION OF THE OXYGEN EQUILIBRIUM CURVE OF HUMAN RED BLOOD CELLS. IN THE ROLE OF STORAGE OF BLOOD ON 2,3-DPG, HEMOGLOBIN-OXYGEN AFFINITY, AND OXYGEN RELEASE WHICH OF THE FOLLOWING WERE OBSERVED?:
A. Blood stored in acid-citrate dextrose rapidly changes its oxygen affinity because of the prompt fall in 2,3-DPG
B. Transfusions of blood low in 2,3-DPC produces a fall in the red cell 2,3-DPG of the recipient
C. Bloods "less than 5 days old" are quite dissimilar because blood stored for only one day has a lower oxygen affinity than does blood stored for 5 days
D. A shift to the left occurs after transfusion with blood which is low in 2,3-DPG in the oxygen equilibrium curve which is accompanied by a fall in the central venous oxygen tension
E. Blood less than 24 hours old appears to be preferable for sick infants with the potential for hypoxemia
Ref. J Pediatr
79:898, December 1971

COMPLICATIONS OF INTRAUTERINE TRANSFUSIONS

88. THE TREATMENT OF Rh SENSITIZATION BY THE TECHNIQUE OF INTRAUTERINE TRANSFUSION HAS RESULTED IN WHICH OF THE FOLLOWING COMPLICATIONS?:
A. Maternal and fetal homologous serum hepatitis
B. Premature labor
C. Amnionitis
D. Death from excessive volumes of low pH A. C. D. donor blood given at a rapid rate
E. Omental herniation

Ref. J Pediatr Surg 7:62, February, 1972
Pediatrics, 45:576, 1970

ERYTHROBLASTOSIS AND CARDIORESPIRATORY STATUS

89. WHICH OF THE FOLLOWING MOST COMMONLY INFLUENCE THE MORTALITY OF PREMATURE INFANTS WHO ARE TREATED FOR SEVERE ERYTHROBLASTOSIS FETALIS?:
A. Asphyxia and acidemia
B. Hypoglycemia
C. Hyaline membrane disease
D. Congestive heart failure
E. Hyperbilirubinemia

Ref. Pediatrics 49:5, January, 1972

ERYTHROCYTE HYDROGEN PEROXIDE HEMOLYSIS TEST

90. THE LABORATORY DIFFERENTIATION OF NEONATAL HEPATITIS AND BILIARY ATRESIA IS OFTEN INCONCLUSIVE, AND EXPLORATORY LAPAROTOMY AND OPERATIVE CHOLANGIOGRAPHY ARE UTILIZED FREQUENTLY TO ESTABLISH THE PATENCY OF THE BILIARY DUCTS. IN UTILIZING THE RED CELL PEROXIDE HEMOLYSIS TEST (PHT) IN THE DIFFERENTIAL DIAGNOSIS OF OBSTRUCTIVE JAUNDICE WHICH OF THE FOLLOWING ARE CORRECT?:
A. When red cells deficient in vitamin E are incubated with H_2O_2, hemolysis occurs
B. Congenital biliary obstruction with absent bile salt excretion leads to deficient red cell membrane vitamin E
C. PHT cannot be used in premature infants to detect liver disease
D. A normal PHT rules out biliary atresia
E. A markedly abnormal PHT is consistent with biliary atresia or the completely obstructive phase of neonatal hepatitis

Ref. Pediatrics 48:562, October, 1971

EXCHANGE TRANSFUSION, REPEAT

91. THE "LATE" POSTEXCHANGE REBOUND IN BILIRUBIN HAS BEEN STUDIED BY MEASURING THE RATE OF HEME TURNOVER AS REFLECTED BY ENDOGENOUS CARBON MONOXIDE PRODUCTION. WHICH OF THE FOLLOWING MECHANISMS MAY EXPLAIN THE INCREASED LEVEL OF HEME CATABOLISM AFTER EXCHANGE TRANSFUSION?:
A. Release of pools of sensitized RBC's from the bone marrow and spleen
B. Continued production of RBC's by bone marrow
C. "Push-pull" technique of exchange transfusion and mechanical damage to RBC's
D. Decreased hepatic clearance
E. "Early-labeled" peak of bilirubin from heme turnover in bone marrow and liver

Ref. Clin. Res 19:208, 1971

INTRA-UTERINE TRANSFUSIONS

92. IN A STUDY OF THE DEVELOPMENT OF 24 NONHYDROPIC FETUSES WHO RECEIVED INTRA-UTERINE TRANSFUSIONS FOR SEVERE ERYTHROBLASTOSIS, AND WHO SURVIVED THE NEONATAL PERIOD, WHICH OF THE FOLLOWING WERE OBSERVED?:
A. High incidence of deafness
B. Normal growth patterns
C. High incidence of spastic paraplegia
D. Lag in expressive language skills
E. Salvage of fetuses who had suffered severe brain damage in utero

Ref. Pediatrics
47:689, 1971

LEUKEMIA AND INFECTION

93. INFECTION HAS BECOME THE MAJOR CAUSE OF DEATH IN CHILDREN WITH LEUKEMIA. WHICH OF THE FOLLOWING OBSERVATIONS PROVIDE A USEFUL APPROACH TO THE DIAGNOSIS AND MANAGEMENT OF INFECTIOUS COMPLICATIONS OF LEUKEMIA?:
A. An absolute neutrophil count of less than 500/ cu mm often heralds a serious infection
B. Pneumocystis carinii pneumonitis occurs most frequently with patients in remission
C. Fever should be considered to be of infectious etiology until proven otherwise
D. Organisms of low virulence rarely cause serious infections in children with acute leukemia
E. Disseminated mycoses continue to be a rare event in children under therapy

Ref. Am J Dis Child
122:283, October, 1971

NITROBLUE TETRAZOLIUM DYE TEST IN FEBRILE DISORDERS

94. IN THE USE OF THE NITROBLUE TETRAZOLIUM DYE TEST (NBT) IN THE LABORATORY DIAGNOSIS OF BACTERIAL AND NONBACTERIAL FEBRILE ILLNESSES, WHICH OF THE FOLLOWING OBSERVATIONS HAVE BEEN MADE?:
A. The NBT test is less reliable than the total and differential white blood cell count
B. The NBT test cannot be utilized as an aid in diagnosis in newborn infants
C. Cellular and humoral mechanisms need not be intact to lend validity to the NBT dye test
D. False positive NBT tests in the normal newborn are related to the increased metabolic activity of the leukocytes
E. The NBT dye test has been particularly useful in sickle cell disease because of the lack of false negative results

Ref. J Pediatr
79:943, December, 1971

PLATELET TRANSFUSIONS

95. CURRENT PLATELET PREPARATIONS FOR TRANSFUSIONS MAY BE CONTAMINATED WITH RED BLOOD CELLS. WHICH OF THE FOLLOWING CONSIDERATIONS SHOULD BE CONSIDERED IN REGARD TO PLATELET TRANSFUSIONS?:
A. ABO antigens are probably present on platelets
B. There is no difference in survival of Rh-positive and Rh-negative platelets given to Rh-negative patients
C. Rh antigens are not present on platelets
D. Rh-negative patients who are receiving immunosuppression may be given platelets from Rh-positive donors with little likelihood of isoimmunization
E. Female patients with less serious illnesses requiring platelet transfusion should receive donations from Rh-negative individuals to avoid sensitization

Ref. N Engl J Med
284:942, April 29, 1971

SICKLE CELL DISEASE AND THE HEMOLYTIC CRISIS

96. HEMOLYTIC CRISES IN SICKLE CELL DISEASE SHOULD SUGGEST WHICH OF THE FOLLOWING DIAGNOSTIC POSSIBILITIES AND PROVOCATIVE STATES?:
A. Infection
B. Acidosis
C. Hypoxia
D. Dehydration
E. G-6-PD deficiency (glucose-6-phosphate dehydrogenase)

Ref. J Pediatr
74:544, April, 1969

SICKLE CELL DISEASE--APLASTIC CRISES

97. AN APLASTIC CRISIS IN A CHILD WITH SICKLE CELL DISEASE MAY THREATEN HIS LIFE AND IS USUALLY ASSOCIATED WITH WHICH OF THE FOLLOWING?:
A. Viral infections are usually associated with aplastic crises
B. Aplastic crises may occur in several members of the family
C. Platelet and white blood cell counts are not usually affected
D. Erythroid aplasia usually terminates spontaneously after 7 to 10 days
E. Transfusions of very fresh packed red cells should be used to insure normal levels of 2, 3, diphosphoglyceride

Ref. Pediatrics
48:629, October, 1971

SICKLE CELL DISEASE

98. DESPITE THE PRESENCE OF SPLENOMEGALY, WHICH OF THE FOLLOWING SUGGEST THAT A CHILD WITH SICKLE CELL DISEASE HAS UNDERGONE "FUNCTIONAL ASPLENIA" AS THE RESULT OF THE VASO-OCCLUSIVE EPISODES?:
   A. Increased susceptibility to serious pneumococcal infections
   B. Presence of Howell-Jolly bodies on peripheral blood smear
   C. Diminished resistance to infection with Salmonella, often localized in bone
   D. Thrombocytopenia
   E. Staphylococcal abscesses in lymph nodes and deep viscera

Ref. Pediatrics
48:631, October, 1971

THALASSEMIA

99. IN A STUDY OF 138 CONSECUTIVE CASES OF COOLEY'S ANEMIA (HOMOZYGOUS BETA-THALASSEMIA), WHICH OF THE FOLLOWING FINDINGS WERE PRESENT IN MOST CHILDREN?:
   A. Cephalofacial deformities
   B. Hepatomegaly
   C. Severe retardation of physical growth
   D. Normal intelligence quotients
   E. Depression and floating anxiety

Ref. Pediatrics
48:740, November, 1971

VITAMIN K

100. IN CLINICAL PROBLEMS WHERE BLEEDING IS RELATED TO HYPOPROTHROMBINEMIA,WHICH OF THE FOLLOWING STATEMENTS ARE CORRECT?:
   A. If the hypoprothrombinemia is responsive to vitamin K bleeding is controlled within a hour
   B. Unresponsiveness to vitamin K may be due to hepatic immaturity in infants
   C. Infants with severe hepatocellular disease may not respond to parenteral vitamin K
   D. Doses of vitamin K larger than 1.0 mg subcutaneously may be necessary in children who do not respond initially to this recommended dose
   E. Intravenous vitamin K may be more effective than its subcutaneous or intramuscular injection

Ref. Pediatrics
48:485, September, 1971

QUESTIONS 101 TO 109 LIST DATA RELATED TO BLEEDING CHILDREN. FOR EACH QUESTION, CHOOSE THE BEST DIAGNOSIS FROM THE LETTERED CHOICES ON THE OPPOSITE PAGE:

NINE BLEEDING CHILDREN

QUESTIONS:	**101**	**102**	**103**	**104**	**105**	**106**	**107**	**108**	**109**
Age (years)	4 days	7	3	4	2	8	6	10	7
Sex	F	M	M	M	F	F	M	F	M
Petechiae	0	0	+	+	0	0	+	0	+
Hemarthrosis	0	+	0	0	0	0	0	0	0
↑ Liver	0	0	0	+	0	0	0	0	0
↑ Spleen	0	0	0	+	+	0	0	0	0
↑ Nodes	0	0	0	0	0	0	0	0	0
Platelets/mm^3 (10^3)	190.	240.	272.	40.	110.	310.	5.	52.	240.
Hb (Gms%)	13.2	12.2	13.0	8.1	11.4	13.8	12.7	23.0	13.4
RBC morphology	N	N	N	Burr Cells	N	N	N	N	N
Tourniquet Test	N	N	+	+	N	N	+	N	N
Bleeding Time (min.) (N:2-10)	6	5	17	12	3	17	12	8	7
Pro. Time (sec.) (N:12-14)	55	13	12	32	45	14	12	22	12
P.T.T. (sec.) (N:34-46)	98	75	41	67	82	51	37	58	40
Bone Marrow (megakaryo.)	–	–	–	↑	–	–	↑	N	–
Clot retraction	↓	↓	↓	↓	N	N	↓	N	–
Thromboplastin Generation Time – plasma defect	0	+	0	+	0	+	0	–	–
serum defect	+	0	0	0	+	0	0	–	–
DIAGNOSIS:									

Courtesy of: J. Lawrence Naiman, M.D., Chief of Pediatric Hematology, St. Christopher's Hospital for Children, Philadelphia, Pennsylvania.

POSSIBLE DIAGNOSES

A. Von Willebrand's disease
B. Idiopathic thrombocytopenic purpura
C. Classical hemophilia (AHF deficiency)
D. Disseminated intravascular coagulation
E. Purpura fulminans
F. Fulminating meningococcemia
G. Hereditary hemorrhagic telangiectasia
H. Banti's syndrome
I. Hemorrhagic disease of the newborn
J. Hepatic cirrhosis
K. Hereditary afibrinogenemia
L. Fibrin stabilizing factor (XIII) deficiency
M. Functional platelet defect
N. Christmas disease
O. Acute lymphoblastic leukemia
P. Cyanotic congenital heart disease
Q. Salicylate ingestion
R. Primary fibrinolysis
S. Henoch-Schonlein purpura
T. Aplastic anemia

QUESTIONS 110 TO 118 LIST DATA RELATED TO ANEMIC PATIENTS. FOR EACH QUESTION, CHOOSE THE BEST DIAGNOSIS FROM THE LETTERED CHOICES ON THE OPPOSITE PAGE:

NINE PATIENTS WITH ANEMIA

QUESTIONS:	110	111	112	113	114	115	116	117	118
Age (years)	4	12	3	7	6	2	1 day	9	21
Sex	F	M	M	F	M	M	F	M	M
Color	W	N	W	W	N	N	W	W	N
Splenomegaly	+	0	+	0	0	0	+	0	0
Hb (Gms. %)	7.4	8.6	4.0	10.4	6.2	5.1	13.2	3.4	15.4
Hct. (%)	19	25	12	34	18	25	39	11	45
RBC (Millions/mm^3)	2.0	2.6	1.2	5.0	2.0	4.1	3.2	1.0	5.1
Reticulocytes (%)	8.0	9.2	24.0	1.8	9.4	1.8	15.0	0.6	1.2
Spherocytes	+	0	+	0	0	0	+	0	0
Sickle cells	0	+	0	0	0	0	0	0	0
Target cells	0	+	0	+	0	0	0	0	0
Ovalocytes	0	0	0	+	0	0	0	0	0
Burr cells / fragmented forms	0	0	0	0	+	0	0	0	0
Blood type	A+	B+	0+	A⁻	B⁻	0⁻	A+	B+	0+
Direct Coombs	Neg	Neg	Pos	Neg	Neg	Neg	Pos	Neg	Neg
Total Bilirubin (mg%)	3.2	2.7	7.6	0.7	4.2	0.5	17.2	1.6	0.4
Osmotic fragility	↑	↓	↑	↓	N	↓	↑	N	N
Hb A_2 (5) (N < 3.1)	2.5	2.4	2.3	4.1	1.5	1.0	0.3	3.1	2.4
Hb F (%) (N < 2.0)	1.8	10.2	1.4	2.2	0.9	2.2	76	1.1	0.7
Sickle prep.	Neg	Pos	Neg	Neg	Neg	Pos	Neg	Neg	Neg
Hemoglobinuria	0	0	+	0	+	0	0	0	0
DIAGNOSIS:									

Courtesy of: J. Lawrence Naiman, M.D., Chief of Pediatric Hematology, St. Christopher's Hospital for Children, Philadelphia, Pennsylvania.

POSSIBLE DIAGNOSES

A. Acute post-hemorrhagic anemia
B. Hereditary spherocytosis
C. Myelofibrosis
D. ABO incompatibility
E. Glucose-6-phosphate dehydrogenase deficiency
F. Pyruvate kinase deficiency
G. Paroxysmal nocturnal hemoglobinuria
H. Pernicious anemia
I. Thalassemia trait
J. Acute stem cell leukemia
K. Iron deficiency anemia
L. Normal individual
M. Anemia of hepatic cirrhosis
N. Sickle - hemoglobin C disease
O. Sickle - thalassemia
P. Acquired auto-immune hemolytic anemia
Q. Hemolytic - uremic syndrome
R. Idiopathic aplastic anemia
S. Pyridoxine - responsive anemia
T. Thalassemia major

QUESTIONS 119 TO 127 BELOW LIST CLINICAL AND LABORATORY DATA RELATED TO PATIENTS WITH THROMBOCYTOPENIA. FOR EACH QUESTION, CHOOSE THE BEST POSSIBLE DIAGNOSIS FROM THE LETTERED CHOICES ON THE OPPOSITE PAGE:

NINE THROMBOCYTOPENIC CHILDREN

QUESTIONS:	119	120	121	122	123	124	125	126	127
Age (years)	11	1½	4	2	7	12	6	2	4 days
Sex	M	F	F	M	M	F	F	M	F
Petechiae	+	0	+	0	0	+	+	+	+
Epistaxis	0	0	0	0	0	+	+	+	0
Duration of symptoms	1 wk.	–	3 wks.	1 wk.	1 day	2 mo.	4 days	22 mo.	1 day
Drugs	Ampicillin	0	Penicillin	Kaopectate	Iron	Iron, B12	Vit. C	Iron; Penicil.	Penicil. Kanamyc.
Other	Sore throat	Irritable	Pain; Tired	Diarrhea	Hematemesis	Tired	URI	Otitis ×3	Meconium ileus
Fever	+	0	+	0	0	0	0	0	0
Sick?	0	0	+	+	+	+	0	0	+
Jaundice	+	0	0	0	+	0	0	0	+
↑Nodes	+	0	+	0	0	0	0	+	0
Liver (cm.)	1	1	2	1	1	1	1	2	1
Spleen (cm.)	3	1	3	1	5	0	0	2	0
Other	Puffy eyes; rash	Pale	0	↓BP	0	Pale	0	Dry Skin	0
Hb (Gms.%)	12.8	3.7	6.7	5.7	8.2	4.7	9.8	9.7	12.1
WBC × 100	14.3	8.4	7.5	13.1	3.5	2.6	13.2	11.4	9.2
Diff. (%) N/L	14/80	40/50	10/90	60/30	44/44	11/84	70/22	54/37	67/25
RBC morphology	N	Hypochr.	N	Burr cells	Hypochr.	N	N	Hypochr.	Burr cells
Platelets (×1000)	10.	40.	20.	52.	70.	5.	3.	15.	18.
B.M. megakaryocyte	↑	N	↓	↑	N	↓	↑	↑	↑
Urinalysis	Alb+	N	N	Alb++ RBC++	N	N	RBC++	N	Alb+
DIAGNOSIS:									

Courtesy of: J. Lawrence Naiman, M.D., Chief of Pediatric Hematology, St. Christopher's Hospital for Children, Philadelphia, Pennsylvania.

POSSIBLE DIAGNOSES

A. Acute leukemia
B. May-Hegglin anomaly
C. Aplastic anemia
D. Henoch-Schonlein purpura
E. Metastatic neuroblastoma
F. Iron deficiency anemia
G. Systemic lupus erythematosus
H. Neonatal isoimmune thrombocytopenic purpura
I. Thalassemia major
J. Megaloblastic anemia
K. Cirrhosis of the liver
L. Purpura fulminans
M. Overwhelming septicemia
N. Hemolytic-uremic syndrome
O. Von Willebrand's disease
P. Wiskott-Aldrich syndrome
Q. Infectious mononucleosis
R. Hyperthyroidism
S. Disseminated intravascular coagulation
T. Rocky Mountain spotted fever
U. Thrombotic thrombocytopenic purpura
V. Idiopathic thrombocytopenic purpura

FOR EACH OF THE FOLLOWING MULTIPLE CHOICE QUESTIONS, SELECT THE ONE APPROPRIATE ANSWER:

CUTANEOUS FISTULAS OF DENTAL ORIGIN

128. CUTANEOUS FACIAL FISTULAS OF DENTAL ORIGIN ARE OFTEN INCORRECTLY DIAGNOSED AND IMPROPERLY TREATED. EACH OF THE FOLLOWING STATEMENTS IN REGARD TO TOOTH-RELATED DERMAL SINUS TRACTS IS CORRECT, EXCEPT:
A. Dental abscesses in the maxilla tend to drain to the zygomatic or infraorbital areas of the face
B. In children, cutaneous dental fistulas are usually located in the submandibular areas or the center of the chin
C. Routine surgical excision of the sinus tract is necessary to prevent prolonged drainage and scarring
D. Chronic root abscesses often occur in children without pain
E. In children, the affected tooth usually has a large carious lesion and periapical abscess

Ref. J Pediatr
79:51, July, 1971

DENTAL CARIES

129. "BABY-BOTTLE CARIES" IS ONE OF THE MOST COMMONLY MISDIAGNOSED ORAL PROBLEMS IN CHILDREN BETWEEN THE AGES OF 18 AND 36 MONTHS, AND OFTEN MASQUERADES UNDER SUCH DIAGNOSES AS AMELOGENESIS IMPERFECTA OR ENAMEL HYPOPLASIA. EACH OF THE FOLLOWING STATEMENTS IS CORRECT, EXCEPT:
A. The child usually takes a bottle of milk or juice to bed as a pacifier
B. The lesion is rarely if ever observed in children where the community water source contains fluoride
C. The type of nipple has no bearing on the entity
D. The lesion is most pronounced on the smooth surfaces near the gingival crevice
E. The maxillary incisor teeth are the most greatly affected

Ref. Clin Pediatr
10:243, April 1971

DENTAL EXTRACTIONS

130. THE NEED FOR ANTIBIOTIC PROPHYLAXIS IN PEDIATRIC PATIENTS WITH RHEUMATIC OR CONGENITAL VALVULAR HEART DISEASE PRIOR TO DENTAL PROCEDURES IS AN INCOMPLETELY RESOLVED PROBLEM. ALL OF THE FOLLOWING STATEMENTS ARE TRUE, EXCEPT:
A. The extraction of normal teeth in pediatric patients for orthodontic purposes is not associated with bacteremia
B. Bacteremia cannot be demonstrated in adult patients undergoing simple procedures such as cleaning and dental prophylaxis
C. In adult patients bacterial endocarditis can be related to dental manipulations at least 50 per cent of the time
D. The presence of periodontal disease may contribute to the bacteremia which follows dental extractions
E. Children with congenital or rheumatic valvular disease who are undergoing restoration of carious teeth may not need antibiotic prophylaxis

Ref. Amer J Dis Child
121:286, April, 1971

PREMATURE LOSS OF TEETH

131. AN EDENTULOUS 12 YEAR-OLD BOY HAS HYPERKERATOSIS OF THE PALMS AND SOLES AND CALCIFICATION OF THE DURA. HIS DECIDUOUS TEETH WERE LOST AT 5 YEARS, BUT THE ERUPTION OF HIS PERMANENT DENTITION WAS NORMAL. THE MOST LIKELY DIAGNOSIS IS:
A. Hypophosphatasia
B. Hand-Schuller-Christian disease
C. Papillon-Lefevre syndrome
D. Oculo-dento-digital syndrome
E. Ectodermal dysplasia

Ref. N Engl J Med
284:1076, May 13, 1971

PERIODONTAL DESEASE

132. THE TERM PERIODONTAL DISEASE REFERS TO ALL DISEASES OF THE TISSUES SURROUNDING AND SUPPORTING THE TEETH IN THE JAWS. TOGETHER WITH DENTAL CARIES IT REPRESENTS ONE OF THE TWO MOST COMMON ORAL DISEASES OF MAN. EACH OF THE FOLLOWING STATEMENTS IS CORRECT IN REGARD TO PERIODONTAL DISEASE, EXCEPT:
A. Periodontitis is a common and painful disease of neglect in children
B. Gingivitis is the earliest stage of periodontitis
C. In patients with periodontal disease the act of chewing may initiate bacteremia
D. Poor oral hygiene is by far the most important factor responsible for periodontal disease
E. Dental plaque formation is enhanced by the presence of sucrose in the diet

Ref. N Engl J Med
284:1071, May 13, 1971

133. THE PREVALENCE AND SEVERITY OF PERIODONTAL DISEASE INCREASE WITH AGE, AND MUCH RESPONSIBILITY RESTS WITH THE CHILD AND HIS FAMILY IN LEARNING AND PROMOTING PROPER ORAL HYGIENE. EACH OF THE FOLLOWING IS CORRECT, EXCEPT:
A. Malocclusion contributes to the tissue loss of periodontitis
B. Hyperplasia of the gingiva from diphenylhydantoin (Dilantin) does not recur after surgical removal even when the drug is continued
C. Most patients with gingivitis have abnormal ascorbic acid levels
D. Gingival recession and pathologic migration of teeth accompany untreated periodontitis
E. In laboratory animals some forms of periodontitis are transmissible, but no evidence exists in humans for contagiousness

Ref. N Engl J Med
284:1077, May 13, 1971

GENODERMATOSES

THE IMPORTANCE OF A SKIN BIOPSY IN ARRIVING AT A CORRECT DIAGNOSIS IN CERTAIN GENODERMATOSES IS CRUCIAL IN GENETIC COUNSELING. MATCH THE DISORDERS WITH THE CLINICAL CHARACTERISTICS IN THE FOLLOWING ENTITIES IN WHICH A BIOPSY IS EITHER DIAGNOSTIC OR CHARACTERISTIC:

PART A

134. ___ Basal cell nevus syndrome
135. ___ Epidermolysis bullosa, simplex
136. ___ Keratosis follicularis (Darier's)
137. ___ Erythropoietic protoporphyria
138. ___ Lipoid proteinosis

A. Ridging of nails, firm greasy crusted papules progressing to warty plaques, vegetating masses in flexures
B. Enlarged, firm tongue, hoarseness, xanthomatous-like infiltrates on mucous membranes and skin
C. Broad facies, rib anomalies, onset in adolescence, pits on palms, odontogenic cysts of mandible, ectopic calcification of the falx cerebri
D. Photosensitivity, burning, tingling, urticarial lesions, vacciniform vesicles which lead to scarring
E. Intraepidermal blisters induced by trauma, no scarring, onset in infancy

PART B

139. ___ Neurofibromatosis
140. ___ Tuberous sclerosis
141. ___ Incontinentia pigmenti
142. ___ Anhidrotic ectodermal dysplasia
143. ___ Xeroderma pigmentosum

A. CNS abnormalities, hypodontia, vesicular lesions in infancy with eosinophilia
B. Freckling, telangiectasis, early development of basal cell carcinomas
C. Goose-like flesh, periungual fibromata, cardiac and renal hamartomas
D. Axillary freckling, scoliosis, pseudoarthroses, macrodactylia
E. Prominent lips, hypodontia, sparse to absent hair

Ref. Pediatr Clin North Am
18:757, August, 1971

GENODERMATOSES

IN THE FOLLOWING GENODERMATOSES, SKIN BIOPSY IS OF LITTLE OR NO VALUE IN ESTABLISHING A DIAGNOSIS AND IN AIDING IN GENETIC COUNSELING. MATCH THE DISORDER WITH THE CLINICAL CHARACTERISTICS:

PART C

144. ___ Familial angioneurotic edema
145. ___ Hereditary lymphedema (Milroy's)
146. ___ Peutz-Jeghers syndrome
147. ___ Acrodermatitis enteropathica
148. ___ Ataxia telangiectasia

A. Alopecia, diarrhea, vesicular and crusted lesions around orifices and on extremities
B. C'1-esterase inhibitor deficiency, onset usually in early childhood
C. Malignancies of the lymphoreticular system; combined immunologic deficiency disease
D. Intestinal bleeding, intussusception
E. Dilated lymph vessels in dermis and subcutaneous tissue with fibrosis of dermis and fat

PART D

149. ___ Hereditary hemorrhagic telangiectasia (Rendu-Osler-Weber)
150. ___ Chediak-Higashi syndrome
151. ___ Bloom's syndrome
152. ___ Cockayne's syndrome
153. ___ Hartnup's disease

A. Ataxia, aminoaciduria, photosensitivity
B. Premature atherosclerosis, facial erythema in butterfly distribution following light exposure
C. Erythema and telangiectasia of sun-exposed areas; cafe-au-lait spots, death often from malignancy
D. Partial albinism, recurrent infections, large granular inclusions in leukocytes
E. Arterio-venous fistulas in lung, epistaxis, cirrhosis

Ref. Pediatr Clin North Am 18:757, August, 1971

FOR EACH OF THE FOLLOWING MULTIPLE CHOICE QUESTIONS, SELECT THE ONE APPROPRIATE ANSWER:

BULLAE AND THE EOSINOPHIL

154. A COMBINATION OF BULLAE AND LINEAR VERRUCOUS LESIONS ON THE EXTREMITIES OF AN INFANT GIRL WITH A HIGH EOSINOPHIL COUNT TOGETHER WITH DECIDUOUS TEETH WHICH SHOW HYPODONTIA SHOULD SUGGEST:

A. Ectodermal dysplasia
B. Bullous urticaria pigmentosa
C. Dermatitis herpetiformis
D. Incontinentia pigmenti
E. Epidermolysis bullosa

Ref. Am J Dis Child 122:294, October, 1971

PHOTODERMATITIS

155. CONTACT PHOTODERMATITIS USUALLY RESULTS FROM EXPOSURE TO LIGHT IN THE ULTRAVIOLET RANGE OF 280 TO 400 NANOMETERS. EACH OF THE FOLLOWING IS CORRECT, EXCEPT:

A. Some individuals with systemic lupus erythematosus are photosensitive to ultraviolet light
B. Light from an electric (microwave) oven is an unappreciated source for the potential of producing a photodermatitis
C. Photosensitivity is seen in porphyria cutanea tarda
D. Photoreactive substances may be present in deodorant soaps and toiletries (containing halogenated salicylanilides and bithionol)
E. Systemic drugs which have been incriminated in photodermatitis include the tetracyclines

Ref. JAMA
216:1651, June 7, 1971

STAPHYLOCOCCI, PHAGE II

156. PHAGE GROUP II COAGULASE-POSITIVE STAPHYLOCOCCI HAVE BEEN ASSOCIATED WITH ALL OF THE FOLLOWING CUTANEOUS SYNDROMES, EXCEPT:

A. Toxic epidermal necrolysis
B. Ritter's disease (generalized exfoliative disease in infants)
C. Erythema multiforme exudativum
D. Scarlatiniform erythema with exfoliation (staphylococcal scarlet fever)
E. Bullous impetigo

Ref. J Pediatr
78:958, June, 1971
J Infect Dis
125:129, February, 1972

SCALDED SKIN SYNDROME

157. THE DEVELOPMENT OF AN EXPERIMENTAL ANIMAL MODEL CLEARLY ESTABLISHES THE ETIOLOGIC RELATIONSHIP IN TOXIC EPIDERMAL NECROLYSIS WITH THE STAPHYLOCOCCUS. THE CLINICAL PICTURE OF LYELL'S DISEASE PRESENTS ALL OF THE FOLLOWING FEATURES, EXCEPT:

A. Exquisite sensitivity of the skin
B. Positive Nikolsky's sign
C. Increased erythema in the skin creases resembling Pastia's lines
D. Fluid aspirated from bullae may be sterile
E. Beneficial effects of corticosteroid therapy

Ref. J Pediatr
78:965, June, 1971

STAPHYLOCOCCAL SCARLATINIFORM RASH

158. NONSTREPTOCOCCAL SCARLATINIFORM RASHES ASSOCIATED WITH STAPHYLOCOCCAL INFECTIONS RESEMBLE THE EXANTHEM OF STREPTOCOCCAL DISEASE. ALL OF THE FOLLOWING STATEMENTS ARE CORRECT IN REFERENCE TO STAPHYLOCOCCAL "SCARLET FEVER," EXCEPT:

A. A rash which resembles "sunburned sandpaper"
B. Accentuation of erythema in the skin creases
C. Absence of a palatal enanthem or a strawberry tongue
D. Desquamation which is identical in appearance and timing with that seen following streptococcal disease
E. Amelioration of the disease with methicillin therapy

Ref. J Pediatr
78:959, June, 1971

STONY-HARD SKIN

159. A CHILD WITH LOCALIZED AREAS (BUTTOCKS AND UPPER THIGHS) OF STONY-HARD SKIN, MILD HIRSUTISM AND LIMITATION OF JOINT MOBILITY WITHOUT MUCOPOLYSACCHARIDURIA WOULD BE SUSPECTED OF HAVING WHICH OF THE FOLLOWING SYNDROMES?:
A. Scheie's
B. Hurler's
C. Stiff skin
D. Scleroderma
E. Morphea

Ref. Pediatrics
47:360, 1971

SUNLIGHT AND THE SKIN

160. MANY DISEASES AND THEIR ASSOCIATED SKIN MANIFESTATIONS ARE EXACERBATED OR WORSENED BY EXPOSURE TO SUN ALTHOUGH LESIONS USUALLY DEVELOP ONLY IN AREAS THAT HAVE RECEIVED INTENSE LIGHT EXPOSURE. ALL OF THE FOLLOWING CLINICAL ENTITIES MAY BE ADVERSELY AFFECTED BY SUNSHINE, EXCEPT:
A. Herpes simplex
B. Varicella
C. Systemic lupus erythematosus
D. Sarcoid
E. Erythema nodosum

Ref. JAMA
217:1088, August 23, 1971

URTICARIA PIGMENTOSA

161. URTICARIA PIGMENTOSA IS CHARACTERIZED BY ABNORMAL ACCUMULATIONS OF MAST CELLS IN THE SKIN. THIS ENTITY HAS BEEN ASSOCIATED WITH ALL OF THE FOLLOWING CLINICAL AND LABORATORY FEATURES, EXCEPT:
A. Circulating heparin-like anticoagulants
B. Discharge of histamine after the ingestion of aspirin and codeine
C. Improvement or disappearance at puberty
D. Response to antihistamines
E. Reactive hyperpigmentation which may persist for life

Ref. Pediatr Clin North Am
18:733, August, 1971

FOR EACH OF THE FOLLOWING QUESTIONS, SELECT THE ONE MOST APPROPRIATE ANSWER BY USING THE KEY OUTLINED BELOW:
1. If A, B and C are correct
2. If A and C are correct
3. If B and D are correct
4. If all are correct
5. If all are incorrect

ACNE

162. WHICH OF THE FOLLOWING STATEMENTS ARE CORRECT IN REGARD TO ACNE?:
A. Acute papulopustular acne has been related to prolonged intravenous hyperalimentation in which the diet was deficient in cystein, tyrosine and glutamic acid
B. Pustular acne has followed the intramuscular use of large doses of cyanocobalamin
C. The rash of pellagra may mimic comedone acne
D. Pupulopustular acne has been associated with hyperglycemia
E. Scientific evidence exists that acne is worsened by chocolate, nuts and iodine

Ref. JAMA
219:877, February 14, 1972

ACNE AND ANTIBIOTICS

163. IN THE TREATMENT OF ACNE WITH ANTIBIOTICS WHICH OF THE FOLLOWING STATEMENTS ARE CORRECT?:
A. Tetracyclines suppress the production of free fatty acids which are the most irritating components of sebum
B. Improvement occurs in all forms of acne including comedones
C. Antibiotic treatment of acne does not appear to affect existing lesions but rather helps in preventing the formation or reducing the severity of newly developing lesions
D. The anti-lipolytic action of tetracyclines is evident within a few days in all patients
E. The organism most frequently recovered from pustular lesions is coagulase-positive staphylococcus aureus

Ref. Pediatrics
48:663, October, 1971

ALOPECIA

164. WHICH OF THE FOLLOWING AGENTS HAVE BEEN ASSOCIATED WITH TOXIC FOLLICLE-SPECIFIC ALOPECIA?:
A. Cyclophosphamide
B. Methotrexate
C. Thallium
D. Vitamin A
E. Vincristine

Ref. Pediatr Clin North Am
18:969, August, 1971

FOR EACH OF THE FOLLOWING MULTIPLE CHOICE QUESTIONS, SELECT THE ONE APPROPRIATE ANSWER:

CALCITONIN

165. MEDULLARY CARCINOMA OF THE THYROID PROBABLY REPRESENTS A MALIGNANCY OF THE PARAFOLLICULAR OR C CELLS WHICH PRODUCE AND SECRETE CALCITONIN, AND IT IS THEREFORE NOT A NEOPLASM OF "TRUE" THYROID ORIGIN. ALL OF THE FOLLOWING ARE CORRECT IN REGARD TO CALCITONIN, EXCEPT:
A. Calcitonin has hormonal effects which enhance the pharmacophysiology of parathormone
B. Calcium infusions produce a twofold to threefold rise in serum calcitonin in most controls
C. Patients with medullary carcinoma of the thyroid have marked elevations (one to two thousand times) of calcitonin
D. Serum calcitonin levels do not correlate with chronic hypercalcemia or chronic hypocalcemia
E. Calcitonin circulates normally in human serum

Ref. N Engl J Med
283:890, October 22, 1970

GROWTH HORMONE DEFICIENCY

166 PATIENTS WITH ISOLATED GROWTH HORMONE DEFICIENCY SHOW ALL OF THE FOLLOWING CLINICAL CHARACTERISTICS, EXCEPT:
A. Epiphyseal closure follows a normal pattern
B. Pregnancy and lactation may occur in affected women
C. The birth weight and length of affected newborns are normal
D. Hypoglycemia is not an associated problem
E. Isolated growth hormone deficiency may be associated with destructive lesions of the anterior pituitary gland

Ref. Hospital Practice
6:113, February, 1971

GROWTH RETARDATION

167. ALTHOUGH CELL GROWTH HAS BEEN STUDIED BY HISTOLOGIC TECHNIQUES IN THE PAST, NEWER METHODS WHICH INCLUDE THE MEASUREMENT OF TISSUE DESOXYRIBONUCLEIC AND RIBONUCLEIC ACIDS AND OF PROTEIN AND WATER CONTENTS, HAS PERMITTED ACCURATE QUANTITATION OF CELL DIVISION AND ENLARGEMENT. EACH OF THE FOLLOWING IS CORRECT, EXCEPT:
A. Tissue content of desoxyribonucleic acid is an index of cell number
B. Total body muscle mass may be estimated by measurement of the urinary excretion of creatinine
C. Growth hormone is an important regulator of cell division
D. Thyroid hormone is concerned with the control of cell size
E. Cell division in the central nervous system is unaffected by protein-calorie malnutrition

Ref. J Pediatr
78:737, May 1971

GROWTH RETARDATION

168. IN A CHILD WHO IS GROWING IN A CHANNEL AT OR SLIGHTLY BELOW THE THIRD PERCENTILE, WITH A BONE AGE EQUAL TO HIS CHRONOLOGIC AGE, AND WHOSE LINEAR GROWTH VELOCITY IS WITHIN THE NORMAL RANGE, ALL OF THE FOLLOWING MAY BE EXCLUDED WITH THE EXCEPTION OF:
A. Gonadal dysgenesis
B. Protein-calorie malnutrition
C. Endocrinopathies
D. Metabolic diseases
E. Malabsorption syndromes

Ref. J Pediatr
78:740, May, 1971

169. A CHILD IS GROWING IN A CHANNEL SLIGHTLY BELOW, BUT PARALLEL TO THE THIRD PERCENTILE; HIS LINEAR GROWTH VELOCITY IS WITHIN THE LOW NORMAL RANGE. HIS SKELETAL MATURATION IS COMMENSURATE WITH HIS HEIGHT AGE. ALL OF THE FOLLOWING CHARACTERIZE THIS GROWTH PATTERN, EXCEPT:
A. This pattern is characteristic of the child with constitutional delay in growth and development
B. The child's growth potential is adequate
C. Adult height will be achieved at an age later than average
D. Sexual maturation is not delayed
E. The mildly malnourished child persues a similar growth pattern, but his weight tends to be less than average for his height

Ref. J Pediatr
78:740, May, 1971

170. A CHILD IS GROWING IN A CHANNEL WHICH IS RELATIVELY PARALLEL TO, BUT RATHER FAR BELOW, THE THIRD PERCENTILE. HIS LINEAR GROWTH VELOCITY IS AT THE LOWEST LIMITS OF, OR SLIGHTLY BELOW, THE NORMAL RANGE. THE BONE AGE IS SIGNIFICANTLY RETARDED BEHIND THE CHRONOLOGIC AGE AND APPROXIMATELY EQUAL TO THE HEIGHT AGE. ALL OF THE FOLLOWING ARE COMPATIBLE WITH THIS GROWTH PATTERN, EXCEPT:
A. Malnutrition
B. An extreme degree of constitutional delay in growth and development
C. Primary renal tubular acidosis
D. Hypopituitarism
E. A child with genetic short stature who has a limited growth potential

Ref. J Pediatr
78:741, May, 1971

GROWTH RETARDATION

171. A CHILD IS GROWING IN A CHANNEL WHICH PROGRESSIVELY DEVIATES AWAY FROM THE THIRD PERCENTILE OR FROM A PREVIOUSLY RECORDED GROWTH CHANNEL. HIS LINEAR GROWTH VELOCITY IS ABNORMALLY SLOW, AND HIS BONE AGE IS MARKEDLY RETARDED. THIS PATTERN IS CHARACTERISTIC OF A CHILD WITH:
A. Chronic systemic or endocrinologic disease
B. Chondrodystrophies
C. Trisomy 13, 18 and 21
D. Intra-uterine growth retardation associated with placental insufficiency
E. Intra-uterine growth retardation associated with infection such as rubella, toxoplasmosis and cytomegalic inclusion disease

Ref. J Pediatr
78:741, May, 1971

HYPOGONADISM, SECONDARY

172. A 16 YEAR-OLD BOY WITH SHORT STATURE, DELAYED SEXUAL DEVELOPMENT AND ANOSMIA SHOULD BE SUSPECTED OF HAVING:
A. Kallman's syndrome
B. Isolated deficiency of luteinizing hormone
C. Laurence-Moon-Biedl syndrome
D. XYY male
E. XXY Klinefelter's syndrome

Ref. Arch Intern Med
121:534, 1968

HYPOPITUITARISM

173. THE CLINICAL MANIFESTATIONS IN THE CHILD WITH HYPOPITUITARISM ARE USUALLY QUITE DISTINCTIVE. EACH OF THE FOLLOWING IS EXPECTED IN PATIENTS WITH HYPOPITUITARISM WHO DO NOT HAVE DEMONSTRABLE LESIONS OF THE PITUITARY, EXCEPT:
A. The retardation of growth has a variable onset
B. The body proportions are compatible with the retarded height
C. The face is rounded with an immature "doll-like" appearance
D. The genitals may be small even for the size of the patient with a peripelvic distribution of fat
E. The intelligence of pituitary dwarfs is usually below normal

Ref. J Pediatr
78:742, May, 1971

HYPOPITUITARISM

174. IN THE EVALUATION OF PITUITARY FUNCTION IN A CHILD WITH GROWTH FAILURE ALL OF THE FOLLOWING ARE CORRECT, EXCEPT:
A. If growth hormone secretion is abnormal following insulin-induced hypoglycemia the abnormal findings should be confirmed by employing other growth homone-releasing stimuli such as arginine
B. Metyrapone may be employed to study the hypothalamic-pituitary adrenocorticotropin-adrenal axis
C. Secretion of thyrotropin may be assessed indirectly by serum thyroxin concentration and by thyroidal 24 hour I_{131} uptake
D. Luteinizing and follicle-stimulating hormones may be measured in urine by bioassay or radioimmunoassay
E. Peripheral sub or unresponsiveness to growth hormone in children with the clinical manifestations and growth patterns suggestive of hypopituitarism and who have normal or elevated concentrations of growth hormone has not been documented

Ref. J Pediatr
78:743, May, 1971

HYPOTHALAMIC RELEASING HORMONES

175. RELEASING HORMONES FROM THE HYPOTHALAMUS WHICH CONTROL ANTERIOR PITUITARY FUNCTION ARE BECOMING IMPORTANT IN THE DIAGNOSIS OF DISEASES OF THE HYPOTHALAMUS, PITUITARY AND THEIR TARGET ORGANS. WHEN THYROTROPIN-RELEASING HORMONE IS ADMINISTERED WHICH OF THE FOLLOWING IS INCORRECT?:
A. Thyrotropin response with primary thyroid failure is exaggerated and prolonged
B. Absent thyrotropin response in hyperthyroidism
C. All patients who fail to respond are hyperthyroid
D. Increase in the output of prolactin
E. No release of growth hormone or the posterior lobe hormones

Ref. Br Med J
1:65, 1972

ISOSEXUAL PRECOCITY IN THE FEMALE

176. THE MOST UNUSUAL CAUSE OF ISOSEXUAL PRECOCITY IN THE FEMALE IS:
A. Constitutional factors
B. Polyostotic fibrous dysplasia
C. Granulosa cell tumor
D. Adrenal carcinoma
E. Central nervous system lesions

Ref. Modern Medicine
40:68, January 24, 1972

PREPUBERTAL MALE GYNECOMASTIA

177. A 9 YEAR-OLD BOY WHO DEVELOPS BILATERAL BREAST ENLARGEMENT WITH AN INCREASED URINARY EXCRETION OF ESTROGENS AND 17-KETOSTEROIDS SHOULD BE SUSPECTED OF:
A. Adrenal tumor
B. Interstitial cell tumor of the testis
C. Gonadotropin-secreting tumor
D. Exogenous estrogens
E. Idiopathic gynecomastia

Ref. J Pediatr
80:259, February, 1972

SEX CHROMATIN IN THE NEWBORN

178. THE SELECTIVE AFFINITY OF THE Y CHROMOSOME FOR FLUOROCHROME DYES HAS GREATLY AIDED SCREENING NEWBORN INFANTS FOR ABNORMALITIES OF THE SEX CHROMOSOMES. BECAUSE OF ITS CLEAR NUCLEOPLASM, LARGE SIZE AND ELLIPTIC OR ROUND SHAPE WHICH OF THE FOLLOWING TISSUES HAS BEEN FOUND TO BE SUPERIOR TO OTHERS FOR SCREENING FOR ANOMALIES OF THE Y CHROMOSOME IN NEONATES?:
A. Wharton's jelly cells
B. Amniotic membranes
C. Buccal smears
D. White blood cells
E. Skin fibroblasts

Ref. J Pediatr
79:305, August, 1971

TESTICULAR FEMINIZATION SYNDROME

179. AS MANY AS ONE TO TWO PER CENT OF FEMALE CHILDREN WITH INGUINAL HERNIAS HAVE THE SYNDROME OF TESTICULAR FEMINIZATION. EACH OF THE FOLLOWING STATEMENTS IN REGARD TO THE TESTICULAR FEMINIZATION SYNDROME IS CORRECT, EXCEPT:
A. Adolescent patients have scanty pubic hair
B. The external genitalia appear normal
C. There is normal growth and breast development
D. The administration of testosterone is not followed by virilization
E. The presence of a cervix by speculum exam does not rule out the testicular feminization syndrome

Ref. Am J Dis Child
117:243, 1969

THYROTOXICOSIS, MATERNAL

180. DISORDERS OF THE THYROID IN THE NEWBORN MAY RESULT FROM THE TREATMENT OF MATERNAL THYROTOXICOSIS DURING PREGNANCY. EACH OF THE FOLLOWING STATEMENTS IS CORRECT, EXCEPT:
   A. In thyrotoxicosis in the mother long-acting thyroid stimulator (LATS) plays no role in the temporary but potentially life-threatening hyperthyroidism which may be present in the newborn
   B. Antithyroid medication administered to a hyperthyroid woman during pregnancy has produced goiter in the newborn
   C. The maternal ingestion of iodide during pregnancy has produced an increased secretion of fetal thyrotropin (TSH)
   D. Cardiomegaly and high output failure in the newborn may be caused by a massive shunt across the vascular bed of the goiter
   E. The administration of thyroid to the infant will suppress secretion of thyrotropin (TSH) and reduce the size of the goiter

Ref. Pediatrics
47:510, 1971

VASOPRESSIN-RESISTANT DIABETES INSIPIDUS

181. HYPERURICEMIA HAS BEEN DESCRIBED IN ADULT PATIENTS WITH VASOPRESSIN-RESISTANT DIABETES INSIPIDUS. EACH OF THE FOLLOWING IS CORRECT IN NEPHROGENIC DIABETES INSIPIDUS, EXCEPT:
   A. The hyperuricemia appears to be secondary to decreased urate clearance by the kidney
   B. The high rate of urine flow appears to lead to dilatation of the renal pelvis and collecting system
   C. The administration of a diuretic is the only satisfactory way of treating the polyuria
   D. Chlorothiazide therapy may aggravate the hyperuricemia but the concomitant administration of allopurinol may keep the serum uric within a normal range
   E. Water diuresis and high concentrations of plasma vasopressin profoundly influence the renal handling of urates

Ref. N Engl J Med
284:1057, May 13, 1971

NEUROENDOCRINE CONTROL

MATCH THE APPROPRIATE ANSWER:

A. Increased plasma corticoids
B. Increased ACTH levels
C. Decreased ACTH levels
D. Increase in both corticoids and ACTH
E. Absent response (both)

IN TESTING THE NEUROENDOCRINE CONTROL SYSTEM IN PRIMARY ADRENAL DISEASE YOU WOULD EXPECT TO MATCH WHICH OF THE FOLLOWING?:

182. ___ Resting state
183. ___ Response to ACTH
184. ___ Response to vasopressin (CRF)
185. ___ Response to piromen or hypoglycemia

IN TESTING THE NEUROENDOCRINE CONTROL SYSTEM IN ADRENAL INSUFFICIENCY SECONDARY TO PITUITARY DISEASE YOU WOULD EXPECT TO MATCH WHICH OF THE FOLLOWING?:

186. ___ Resting state
187. ___ Response to ACTH
188. ___ Response to vasopressin (CRF)
189. ___ Response to piromen or hypoglycemia

IN TESTING THE NEUROENDOCRINE CONTROL SYSTEM IN ADRENAL INSUFFICIENCY SECONDARY TO HYPOTHALAMIC DISEASE YOU WOULD EXPECT TO MATCH WHICH OF THE FOLLOWING?:

190. ___ Resting state
191. ___ Response to ACTH
192. ___ Response to vasopressin (CRF)
193. ___ Response to piromen or hypoglycemia

Ref. Hospital Practice 6:135, November, 1971

HYPERPARATHYROIDISM

THE DIAGNOSIS OF PRIMARY HYPERPARATHYROIDISM IS BASED UPON LABORATORY DATA WHICH AWAITS THE DEVELOPMENT OF A SPECIFIC IMMUNOASSAY FOR PARATHYROID HORMONE. MATCH THE LABORATORY TEST WITH THE EXPECTED FREQUENCY OF ABNORMALITY:

A. Increased frequently (75% or greater)
B. Decreased frequently (75% or greater)
C. Increased occasionally (less than 25%)
D. Decreased occasionally (less than 25%)

194. ___ Ionized calcium concentration
195. ___ Serum phosphorus concentration
196. ___ Phosphate clearance
197. ___ Serum alkaline phosphatase
198. ___ Serum magnesium

Ref. N Engl J Med 285:1008, October 28, 1971

FOR EACH OF THE FOLLOWING QUESTIONS, SELECT THE ONE APPROPRIATE ANSWER BY USING THE KEY OUTLINED BELOW:

1. If A, B and C are correct
2. If A and C are correct
3. If B and D are correct
4. If all are correct
5. If all are incorrect

CUSHING'S SYNDROME, MATERNAL

199. THE EVENTS SURROUNDING PREGNANCY IN CUSHING'S SYNDROME AND THE FINDINGS IN THE NEWBORN INFANTS WHO HAVE BEEN DELIVERED HAVE BEEN CHARACTERIZED BY WHICH OF THE FOLLOWING?:

A. High rate of fetal loss
B. Vascular collapse in infant
C. Hyponatremia and hyperkalemia in infant
D. Early onset of labor
E. Hypoglycemia in infant

Ref. Pediatrics 47:516, 1971

CYCLIC AMP

200. IN 1971 A NOBEL PRIZE WAS AWARDED FOR RESEARCH INTO THE ACTIONS OF CYCLIC AMP (THE NUCLEOTIDE 3', 5'-ADENOSINE MONOPHOSPHATE) WHICH MEDIATES THE FUNCTIONS OF A GREAT VARIETY OF HORMONES WHICH INCLUDE WHICH OF THE FOLLOWING?:
A. Increased release of insulin
B. Increased renin
C. Increased release of ACTH
D. Increased release of thyroid
E. Increased release of growth hormone

Ref. Med World News
12:48, December 10, 1971

GYNECOMASTIA

201. IN A STUDY OF PITUITARY-GONADAL FUNCTION IN IDIOPATHIC PUBERTAL GYNECOMASTIA,WHICH OF THE FOLLOWING HORMONE ASSAYS WERE OBSERVED?:
A. Normal levels of testosterone for age
B. Normal levels of growth hormone
C. Normal levels of luteinizing hormone
D. Increased levels of testosterone
E. Elevated gonadotropins

Ref. J Pediatr
79:1002, December, 1971

HYPOTHYROIDISM AND ELEVATED BUN

202. ELEVATIONS OF UREA NITROGEN HAVE BEEN OBSERVED IN HYPOTHYROIDISM AND HAVE BEEN ASSOCIATED WITH WHICH OF THE FOLLOWING CLINICAL OBSERVATIONS?:
A. Decrease in protein synthesis
B. Decrease in amino acid utilization
C. Most commonly seen in children under two years of age
D. No impairment of urea excretion
E. High correlation with elevations of serum cholesterol

Ref. Pediatrics
48:829, 1971

KLINEFELTER'S SYNDROME

203. ALTHOUGH KLINEFELTER'S SYNDROME (XXY) IS SECOND IN FREQUENCY ONLY TO DOWN'S SYNDROME, THE DIAGNOSIS IS RARELY MADE UNTIL PUBESCENCE OR LATER. WHICH OF THE FOLLOWING SHOULD SUGGEST THE POSSIBILITY AND LEAD TO EARLIER DETECTION?:
A. Small size of testes
B. Dull mentality
C. Decreased upper-to-lower segment ratio of body
D. Small phallus
E. Decreased weight for height

Ref. J Pediatr
80:250, February, 1972

PNEUMOGRAPHY, PELVIC

204. PELVIC PNEUMOGRAPHY WITH THE USE OF NITROUS OXIDE IS HELPFUL IN DIAGNOSING WHICH OF THE FOLLOWING?:
A. Testicular feminization syndrome
B. Polycystic ovary syndrome
C. Gonadal dysgenesis
D. Normal female pelvic structures in intersex problems
E. Ovarian tumors

Ref. J Pediatr 78:779, May, 1971

STEIN-LEVENTHAL SYNDROME

205. IN AN ADOLESCENT GIRL WHO IS COMPLAINING OF HIRSUTISM AND MENSTRUAL IRREGULARITIES, WHICH OF THE FOLLOWING ESTABLISH A DIAGNOSIS OF STEIN-LEVENTHAL SYNDROME OR POLYCYSTIC OVARIES?:
A. Moderate elevations of urinary 17-ketosteroids
B. Pelvic pneumography
C. Elevated plasma testosterone and luteinizing hormone
D. Buccal smear
E. Urinary gonadotropins

Ref. J Pediatr 78:779, May, 1971

FOR EACH OF THE FOLLOWING MULTIPLE CHOICE QUESTIONS, SELECT THE ONE APPROPRIATE ANSWER:

ALPHA 1-ANTITRYPSIN DEFICIENCY

206. IN SOME CHILDREN WITH CIRRHOSIS OF THE LIVER AN INHERITED DEFICIENCY OF AN ANTIENZYME, ALPHA-1-ANTITRYPSIN, HAS BEEN RECENTLY IDENTIFIED. EACH OF THE FOLLOWING OBSERVATIONS IS CORRECT, EXCEPT:

A. The liver is the only organ that produces alpha-1-antitrypsin
B. There is increased accumulation of alpha-1-antitrypsin in the livers of children with familial cirrhosis associated with serum deficiencies of this antienzyme
C. In children affected with this disease electrophoretic patterns in early life may be normal for alpha-1-antitrypsin
D. Trypsin inhibitory capacity determinations in children with hepatic cirrhosis associated with biliary atresia and cystic fibrosis have been normal or above-normal
E. The clinical manifestations of alpha-1- antitrypsin deficiency and hepatic cirrhosis begin in the first year of life

Ref. Hospital Practice
6:83, May, 1971

ATRESIA, ANORECTAL

207. THE SITE OF ATRESIA IN ANORECTAL ANOMALIES IS IMPORTANT TO DOCUMENT IN REGARD TO THE SURGICAL CORRECTION OF THE ANOMALY AS WELL AS IDENTIFYING CONCOMITANT DEFORMITIES OF THE UROGENITAL SYSTEM. IT HAS BEEN SUGGESTED THAT THE MOST ACCURATE AND CONVENIENT METHOD FOR DETERMINING THE LEVEL OF ATRESIA OF THE RECTUM MAY BE:

A. Lateral plain X-ray in the upside-down position
B. Cystogram to show a rectourethral fistula
C. An oral contrast study
D. Contrast filling of the distal loop and pouch of the rectum via a colostomy
E. Ultrasonic-echo examination

Ref. J Pediatr Surg
6:454, August, 1971

BILE-STAINED VOMITUS AND MELENA

208. THE COINCIDENCE OF GREEN BILE-STAINED VOMITING AND THE PASSAGE OF BLOOD PER RECTUM IN THE NEWBORN INFANT SHOULD SUGGEST:

A. Hirschsprung's disease
B. Volvulus
C. Meconium ileus
D. Duplications of the bowel
E. Duodenal atresia

Ref. Progr Pediatr Surg
2:57, 1971

CIRRHOSIS, CHILDHOOD IN INDIA

209. INFANTILE CIRRHOSIS OF THE LIVER IS A MAJOR CAUSE OF DEATH AMONG YOUNG CHILDREN IN INDIA, BURMA AND PAKISTAN. THE DISEASE IS INVARIABLY FATAL AND IS MORE COMMONLY SEEN IN MALES. ALL OF THE FOLLOWING LABORATORY OBSERVATIONS HAVE BEEN MADE, EXCEPT:
A. Low serum complement levels
B. Generalized aminoaciduria
C. Detectable alpha-fetoprotein in about one-third of children
D. Absence in serum of the hepatitis-associated antigen in all cases
E. Elevated immunoglobulins

Ref. Lancet
p. 537, March 14, 1970

CYSTIC FIBROSIS

210. GASTROGRAFIN (SQUIBB, METHYLGLUCAMINE DIAGTRIZOATE) ENEMAS HAVE BEEN USED RECENTLY IN THE TREATMENT OF MECONIUM ILEUS. EACH OF THE FOLLOWING STATEMENTS IS CORRECT, EXCEPT:
A. The meconium in cystic fibrosis patients contains less water than normal meconium
B. The use of Gastrografin by enema may cause marked shifts of fluids and electrolytes into the lumen of the bowel
C. The nonoperative approach to meconium ileus may be used for all infants
D. Meconium may be passed within minutes or up to an hour after the termination of the enema
E. No attempt is necessary to withdraw the Gastrografin which is not expelled by the infant

Ref. J Pediatr Surg
5:649, 1970

CYSTIC FIBROSIS AND INTUSSUSCEPTION

211. INTUSSUSCEPTION IS ONE OF THE LESSER APPRECIATED INTESTINAL COMPLICATIONS OF CYSTIC FIBROSIS AND MAY OCCUR MORE FREQUENTLY THAN COMMONLY THOUGHT. THE JUDICIOUS USE OF THE BARIUM ENEMA AS A MEANS OF REDUCING THE INTUSSUSCEPTION OF CYSTIC FIBROSIS IS SUGGESTED BY ALL OF THE FOLLOWING, EXCEPT:
A. There is a lesser incidence of blood in the stool than in otherwise healthy children with intussusception
B. The large size of the colon as a result of chronic fecal overloading may aid in the reduction
C. There is usually easy reduction of the intussusception at surgery
D. The older age group of the patients and the larger physical size may add to the safety of the enema
E. There is little or no likelihood of recurrence of the intussusception in children with cystic fibrosis

Ref. Pediatrics
48:51, July, 1971

DIARRHEA, ENTEROPATHOGENIC E. COLI

212. THERE IS GROWING EVIDENCE THAT CERTAIN STRAINS OF ESCHERICHIA COLI MAY BE RESPONSIBLE FOR DIARRHEAL DISEASE IN ADULTS AS WELL AS IN CHILDREN. IN EXPERIMENTAL INFECTIONS IN MAN ALL OF THE FOLLOWING HAVE BEEN DEMONSTRATED, EXCEPT:
A. Certain strains of E. coli are capable of penetrating intestinal epithelial cells
B. Strains of E. coli are capable of causing symptoms by the elaboration of an enterotoxin
C. Severe systemic symptoms have accompanied experimental infections
D. Blood cultures are commonly positive
E. No practical laboratory procedure is available to identify enterotoxin producing strains

Ref. N Engl J Med
285:1, July 1, 1971

213. DIARRHEA DUE TO ENTEROPATHOGENIC TYPES OF ESCHERICHIA COLI (EPEC) IS RELATED TO AN EXOTOXIN PRODUCED BY THE ORGANISM WHICH CAUSES MOVEMENT OF ELECTROLYTES AND FLUID ACROSS THE INTESTINAL MUCOSA. ALL OF THE FOLLOWING STATEMENTS ARE CORRECT, EXCEPT:

A. Enteropathogenic E. coli organisms have not been demonstrated to invade the infant through the intestinal mucosa
B. The capacity to produce an enterotoxin can be transmitted from one strain of E. coli to another and to other species of bacteria by sexual conjugation
C. Diarrheal disease is almost unknown in newborn infants in primitive cultures even when the baby is delivered and cared for in the filthiest of circumstances
D. A few strains of pseudomonas have recently been found to produce an enterotoxin and may at times be responsible for "diarrhea of unknown etiology"
E. Gentamicin has proven to be an excellent drug in the treatment of EPEC disease and bacterial resistance has not been demonstrated as yet

Ref. J Pediatr
79:8, July, 1971

ENTEROCOLITIS, NECROTIZING

214. THE SYNDROME OF NEONATAL NECROTIZING ENTEROCOLITIS IS RECEIVING GROWING RECOGNITION, AND EACH OF THE FOLLOWING STATEMENTS ARE CORRECT CONCERNING THIS CLINICAL ENTITY, EXCEPT:

A. It is most commonly seen in a stressed and ill premature infant
B. It has not been reported in breast-fed infants
C. There is no evidence that necrotizing enterocolitis is contagious
D. Strictures of the bowel have been reported in survivors
E. A search for a specific infectious agent has been fruitless

Ref. Pediatrics
48:345, September, 1971

ENTEROKINASE DEFICIENCY

215. DEFICIENCY OF INTESTINAL ENTEROKINASE IS ASSOCIATED WITH ALL OF THE FOLLOWING, EXCEPT:

A. Malabsorption and hypoproteinemia
B. Growth failure
C. Abnormal pancreatic secretion
D. Low proteolytic activity in duodenal juice
E. Improvement with protein hydrolysates

Ref. J Pediatr
78:481-490, March, 1971

ESOPHAGEAL ATRESIA

216. BASED UPON EXPERIENCE IN OVER 300 NEWBORN INFANTS WITH ESOPHAGEAL ATRESIA THE RADIOLOGIC DIAGNOSIS IS BEST MADE WITH THE USE OF:

A. Ordinary red rubber catheter
B. Gastrografin
C. Water-soluble iodine mixture
D. Thin barium-water mixture
E. Iodized oil

Ref. Progr Pediatr Surg
2:41, 1971

FOREIGN BODIES IN THE GI TRACT

217. THE MOST COMMON SITE FOR THE IMPACTION OF FOREIGN BODIES IN THE GASTROINTESTINAL TRACT IS:
A. Esophagus
B. Pylorus
C. Duodenum
D. Duodenojejunal flexure
E. Ileocecal region

Ref. Br Med J
4:469, November 20, 1971

218. THE MOST COMMON SITE FOR THE PERFORATION OF FOREIGN BODIES IN THE GASTROINTESTINAL TRACT IS:
A. Esophagus
B. Pylorus
C. Duodenum
D. Duodenojejunal flexure
E. Ileocecal region

Ref. Br Med J
4:46, 1971

GLUTEN ENTEROPATHY

219. GLUTEN-INDUCED ENTEROPATHY IS A DISEASE OF UNKNOWN ETIOLOGY IN WHICH INTESTINAL MALABSORPTION IS PROVOKED BY THE INTERACTION OF ALL OF THE FOLLOWING GLUTENS WITH THE MUCOSA OF THE SMALL INTESTINE, EXCEPT:
A. Oat
B. Rye
C. Corn
D. Wheat
E. Barley

Ref. N Engl J Med
285:1470, December 23, 1971

CHRONIC HEPATITIS

220. THE SUSCEPTIBILITY TO PERSISTENT AUSTRALIAN-ANTIGEN IN SERUM APPEARS TO BE IN THE ORDER OF 3 TO 4 PER CENT OF THE GENERAL POPULATION. THE RISK OF DEVELOPING CHRONIC HEPATITIS IN PATIENTS WITH PERSISTENT AU-ANTIGEN POSITIVE SERUM APPEARS TO BE BEST CORRELATED WITH:
A. Previous acute hepatitis associated with Au-antigen
B. Down's syndrome
C. Healthy carriers
D. All of the above
E. None of the above

Ref. N Engl J Med
285:1159, November 18, 1971

HIRSCHSPRUNG'S DISEASE IN NEWBORNS AND INFANTS

221. CONGENITAL AGANGLIONOSIS OF THE COLON IS THE MOST COMMON CONGENITAL, NONMECHANICAL CAUSE OF INTESTINAL OBSTRUCTION. HIRSCHSPRUNG'S DISEASE IS CHARACTERIZED BY ALL OF THE FOLLOWING, EXCEPT:

A. The distal narrow segment can become passively dilated by impacted stool and repeated enemas and manipulations of the rectum
B. Large irregular saw-toothed contractions are often visualized by X-ray in the aganglionic segment
C. The disease has a significant relationship to congenital heart disease and mongolism
D. Abdominal distention, constipation and absence of diarrhea are seen in all patients
E. Barium retention freely distrubuted throughout the colon proximal to the aganglionic segment 24 to 48 hours after the barium enema is highly suggestive of Hirschsprung's disease in newborn infants

Ref. Clin Pediatr
10:227, April, 1971

INTESTINAL LYMPHANGIECTASIA

222. MORE THAN FORTY DIFFERENT ENTITIES HAVE BEEN ASSOCIATED WITH A PROTEIN-LOSING ENTEROPATHY. DILATATION OF THE SMALL INTESTINAL LYMPHATICS (LYMPHANGIECTASIA) HAS BEEN A FREQUENT FINDING IN MANY OF THE PATIENTS WITH THIS SYNDROME. EACH OF THE FOLLOWING STATEMENTS REGARDING INTESTINAL LYMPHANGIECTASIA IS CORRECT, EXCEPT:

A. There has not been an increased incidence of infection in these children
B. Massive fat excretion in the stools is the rule
C. $Alpha_2$ macroglobulin and fibrinogen levels are unaffected although hypoproteinemia is regularly seen
D. Lymphopenia is a hallmark of the disease
E. D-xylose absorption is characteristically normal

Ref. Arch Dis Childhood
44:527, August, 1969

INTESTINAL PERFORATION IN THE NEWBORN

223. THE ILEUM IS THE MOST VULNERABLE SECTION OF THE GUT IN THE NEWBORN TO IRREVERSIBLE ISCHEMIA. PERFORATIONS OF THE ILEUM HAVE HAD AN ASSOCIATION WITH ALL OF THE FOLLOWING CLINICAL PROBLEMS, EXCEPT:

A. Placenta praevia
B. Exchange transfusion
C. Severe hypothermia
D. Maternal toxemia
E. Maternal diabetes

Ref. Clin Pediatr
10:30, January, 1971

LACTASE DEFICIENCY IN ORIENTALS

224. THE USE OF LACTOSE-CONTAINING FOODS, I.E., DRIED SKIMMED MILK, IN NUTRITIONAL SUPPLEMENTATION PROGRAMS MAY BE CONTRAINDICATED IN VARIOUS RACES LIVING IN DIFFERENT PARTS OF THE WORLD. EACH OF THE FOLLOWING IS CORRECT EXCEPT:
A. Studies in various populations have shown an apparently higher incidence of lactase deficiency in persons of oriental extraction and in Negroes
B. Attempts to increase tolerance to milk products among lactase deficient adults by increased consumption have failed in clinical studies
C. It is unusual for lactase deficiency to persist for more than a few weeks after diarrheal disease
D. Clinical evidence suggests that lactase deficiency may be associated with protein-calorie malnutrition
E. Lactose tolerance tests have been shown to be a useful screening procedure for determining lactase deficiency

Ref. J Pediatr
78:710, April, 1971

PORTAL VENOUS GAS

225. THE PRESENCE OF GAS IN THE PORTAL VENOUS SYSTEM IS A SERIOUS PROGNOSTIC SIGN. THE SURVIVAL IN INFANTS HAS BEEN GREATEST IN WHICH OF THE FOLLOWING ENTITIES WHICH HAVE BEEN ASSOCIATED WITH THIS COMPLICATION?:
A. Hydrogen peroxide enema
B. Umbilical vein catheterization
C. Sepsis
D. Necrotizing enterocolitis in prematures
E. Gastroenteritis

Ref. J Pediatr
79:255, August, 1971

REYE'S SYNDROME

226. THE LEAST TYPICAL CLINICAL FEATURE OF REYE'S SYNDROME IS:
A. Hypoglycemia
B. Elevated blood ammonia
C. Hyperbilirubinemia
D. Hepatomegaly
E. Acidosis

Ref. N Engl J Med
286:257, February 3, 1972

SCHWACHMAN SYNDROME

227. THE MOST FREQUENT FORM OF EXOCRINE PANCREATIC INSUFFICIENCY IN INFANTS AND CHILDREN AFTER CYSTIC FIBROSIS APPEARS TO BE THE SCHWACHMAN SYNDROME. EACH OF THE FOLLOWING STATEMENTS IN REGARD TO THE SCHWACHMAN SYNDROME IS CORRECT, EXCEPT:
A. Growth failure is an inconstant feature
B. Metaphyseal dysostosis is occasionally seen
C. Neutropenia is a regular finding and is unaffected by the administration of pancreatic enzyme supplements
D. The children have normal sweat electrolytes
E. 25 per cent of the published cases have died in infancy or during childhood

Ref. Helvetica Paediatrica Acta
24:547, December, 1969

TRAUMA, SMALL BOWEL

228. INJURIES TO THE SMALL BOWEL FOLLOWING BLUNT ABDOMINAL TRAUMA IN CHILDREN ARE MORE COMMON THAN GENERALLY APPRECIATED. ALL OF THE FOLLOWING ARE CORRECT, EXCEPT:
A. Injuries are most common in the duodenum and proximal jejunum where the bowel is relatively fixed
B. Mesenteric avulsion is the most common complication of small bowel injury in children
C. Duodenal intramural hematomas may be associated with obstruction
D. Over 50 per cent of duodenal intramural hematomas resolve with conservative management
E. The key to diagnosis of small bowel injury in children is repeated physical examination since roentgenograms have limitations

Ref. Pediatr Dig
13:25, July, 1971

CHRONIC ULCERATIVE COLITIS

229. IN CHRONIC ULCERATIVE COLITIS AT THE TIME OF INITIAL DIAGNOSIS, ALL OF THE FOLLOWING HAVE BEEN ASSOCIATED WITH A HIGH RISK OF CANCER, EXCEPT:
A. The first ten years of the disease
B. A clinically severe first attack
C. Continuous rather than intermittent symptoms
D. Universal involvement of the colon
E. Onset of the disease in childhood

Ref. N Engl J Med
285:50, July 1, 1971

230. AT PRESENT, THE BEST CHANCE OF IMPROVING THE LONG-TERM PROGNOSIS OF CHILDREN WITH ULCERATIVE COLITIS APPEARS TO REST WITH:
A. Corticosteroids, orally and by rectum
B. Radical surgery
C. Ileostomy
D. Salicylazosulfapyridine (Azulfidine)
E. Corticosteroids and psychotherapy

Ref. N Engl J Med
285:17, July 1, 1971

VIRAL HEPATITIS AND ARTHRITIS

231. A SIGNIFICANT PERCENTAGE OF PATIENTS WITH BOTH INFECTIOUS AND SERUM HEPATITIS HAVE ARTHRITIS OR ARTHRALGIA WHICH ADDS TO THE DIAGNOSTIC POSSIBILITIES IN A CHILD WITH BOTH HEPATIC AND JOINT DISEASE. ALTHOUGH THE EXPLANATION FOR THE ARTHRITIS IS NOT CLEAR EACH OF THE FOLLOWING IS CORRECT, EXCEPT:
A. Experimental injections of bilirubin products and bile salts have reproduced the syndrome
B. The Australia antigen has been recovered from joint fluid
C. Some children have had decreased levels of complement in both serum and joint fluid
D. The arthritis may involve several joints for weeks and may closely stimulate rheumatoid arthritis
E. The arthritis occurs during the prodome and disappears as clinical evidence of hepatitis appears

Ref. J Pediatr
79:139, July, 1971

FOR EACH OF THE FOLLOWING QUESTIONS, SELECT THE ONE APPROPRIATE ANSWER BY USING THE KEY OUTLINED BELOW:

1. If A, B and C are correct
2. If A and C are correct
3. If B and D are correct
4. If all are correct
5. If all are incorrect

AGANGLIONOSIS

232. WHICH OF THE FOLLOWING VARIATIONS IN PRESENTATION CONTRIBUTE TO THE PITFALLS IN THE EARLY DIAGNOSIS AND TREATMENT OF AGANGLIONIC MEGACOLON?:

A. Enterocolitis
B. Meconium plug syndrome
C. Intestinal obstruction
D. Intestinal perforation
E. Retention of barium-enema in a 24-hour post-evacuation film

Ref. Arch Surg
102:332, April, 1971

ANUS, IMPERFORATE

233. THE EASE OF SURGICAL REPAIR AND BETTER FUNCTIONAL RESULT MAKE IT CRUCIAL TO DISTINGUISH LOW IMPERFORATE ANUS FROM HIGH POUCH ANOMALIES. LOW IMPERFORATE ANUS HAS AN ASSOCIATION WITH WHICH OF THE FOLLOWING?:

A. Male infants with a perineal fistula
B. Male infants with a urethral fistula
C. A blind rectal pouch which lies below the pubococcygeal line
D. A blind rectal pouch which lies outside the puborrectalis sling
E. Male infants with a bladder fistula

Ref. Amer J Dis Child
123:26, January, 1972

CYSTIC FIBROSIS (HERNIAS, HYDROCELES, ETC.)

234. STERILITY IS ALMOST UNIVERSAL IN MALES WITH CYSTIC FIBROSIS. WHICH OF THE FOLLOWING DEFECTS IS SEEN WITH INCREASED FREQUENTLY IN THIS DISEASE?:

A. Inguinal hernia
B. Hydrocele
C. Undescended testicle
D. Congenital absence of the vasa deferentia
E. Anomalous development of the epididymides and seminal vesicles

Ref. Pediatrics
48:442, September, 1971

ESOPHAGEAL ATRESIA

235. ONE OF THE GREATEST ADVANCES IN THE APPROACH TO ESOPHAGEAL ATRESIA HAS BEEN THE STAGING OF SURGICAL PROCEDURES OVER A PERIOD OF TIME. NEARLY ONE-HALF OF INFANTS SHOULD BE STAGED BECAUSE OF WHICH OF THE FOLLOWING?:

A. Prematurity
B. Respiratory distress syndrome
C. Associated major anomalies
D. Wide gap between esophageal segments
E. Small lower segment

Ref. Prog Pediatr Surg
2:41, 1971

ESOPHAGEAL BURNS

236. IN A SUMMARY OF 285 CHILDREN WHO SUSTAINED ACUTE CORROSIVE BURNS OF THE ESOPHAGUS, WHICH OF THE FOLLOWING CONCLUSIONS WERE REACHED?:

A. The most common cause of serious esophageal burns in children is sodium hydroxide
B. Strong acids are more likely to cause damage to the stomach and duodenum
C. Esophagoscopy should be carried out as soon as possible
D. Serious esophageal burns may be sustained without oral injury
E. Immediate steroid-antibiotic therapy appears to have decreased the incidence of strictures

Ref. J Pediatr Surg
6:579, October, 1971

HEPATIC NECROSIS

237. ACUTE MASSIVE HEPATIC NECROSIS IN CHILDREN IS MOST APT TO BE ASSOCIATED WITH WHICH OF THE FOLLOWING?:

A. Acute viral hepatitis
B. Halothane
C. Iproniazid
D. Coxsackie virus
E. Cytomegalovirus

Ref. N Engl J Med
286:260, February 3, 1972

PERITONITIS, PRIMARY

238. THE CLINICAL PICTURE OF PRIMARY PERITONITIS OF CHILDHOOD HAS CHANGED SIGNIFICANTLY IN THE PAST 15 TO 20 YEARS AND HAS SHOWN WHICH OF THE FOLLOWING FEATURES?:

A. Hemolytic streptococci have supplanted pneumococci as the predominant bacterial invaders of the peritoneum
B. Viruses have been identified as causative agents in some cases including the rubella virus
C. Diagnostic paracentesis is recommended as of special value in neonates and nephrotics
D. Concurrent appendectomy is contraindicated in those patients undergoing emergency exploration
E. The route of infection in girls appears to be an ascending genital extension from an associated vaginitis

Ref. Australian Pediatr J
7:73, June, 1971

POLYPS, COLON

239. SINCE THE ASSOCIATION OF A JUVENILE POLYP AND AN ADENOMATOUS POLYP IN THE SAME PATIENT HAS NOT BEEN RECORDED, IN WHICH OF THE FOLLOWING SITUATIONS IS THE SURGICAL REMOVAL OF JUVENILE POLYPS OF THE COLON INDICATED?:

A. Repeated blood loss
B. Removal in the second decade if there is a family history of polyposis
C. Removal in the second decade if there are multiple polyps beyond the reach of a sigmoidoscope
D. Removal in the first decade of polyps in the proximal colon
E. Removal of a colon polyp with documented juvenile polyps of the rectum

Ref. Surgery
69:288, February, 1971

ULCERATIVE COLITIS IN INFANCY

240. ULCERATIVE COLITIS IS BEING RECOGNIZED WITH INCREASING FREQUENCY IN INFANTS UNDER ONE YEAR ALTHOUGH IT IS STILL A RARE DISEASE IN THIS AGE GROUP. WHICH OF THE FOLLOWING FINDINGS ARE USUALLY SEEN WITH THIS SERIOUS DISEASE IN INFANCY?:

A. Bloody mucoid diarrhea
B. Arthralgia
C. Friable, edematous and hyperemic mucosa on sigmoidoscopy
D. Pseudopolyps
E. Mucosal ulceration

Ref. J Pediatr Surg 6:264, June, 1971

BIOPSY, SMALL BOWEL

PERORAL BIOPSY OF THE SMALL INTESTINE CONTRIBUTES TO THE DIAGNOSIS OF DIFFUSE DISEASES OF THE MUCOSA OF THE SMALL INTESTINE. MATCH THE DIAGNOSTIC VALUE OF A BIOPSY WITH THE FOLLOWING DISEASES:

A. Biopsy invariably of diagnostic value
B. Biopsy may or may not be of specific diagnostic value
C. Biopsy may be abnormal but not diagnostic
D. Biopsy is normal

241. ___ Regional enteritis
242. ___ Agammaglobulinemia
243. ___ Hypogammaglobulinemia and dysgammaglobulinemia
244. ___ Tropical sprue
245. ___ Gluten-induced enteropathy
246. ___ Pancreatic exocrine insufficiency
247. ___ Abetalipoproteinemia
248. ___ Intestinal lymphangiectasia
249. ___ Vitamin B_{12} deficiency
250. ___ Functional bowel disease (irritable-colon syndrome, chronic nonspecific diarrhea)

Ref. N Engl J Med 285:1470, December 23, 1971

MECONIUM OBSTRUCTION

MATCH THE CORRECT ANSWER WITH THE DIAGNOSTIC FEATURE WHICH AIDS IN DIFFERENTIATING MECONIUM ILEUS FROM THE MECONIUM PLUG SYNDROME IN THE NEWBORN INFANT:

A. Meconium ileus
B. Meconium plug syndrome
C. Both
D. Neither

251. ___ Abnormal meconium
252. ___ Obstruction in small intestine
253. ___ Fecal trypsin absent
254. ___ Association with Hirschsprung's disease
255. ___ Normal absorption studies
256. ___ Scrotal calcifications

Ref. Progr Pediatr Surg 2:57, 1971

FOR EACH OF THE FOLLOWING MULTIPLE CHOICE QUESTIONS, SELECT THE ONE APPROPRIATE ANSWER:

BACTERIURIA, RECURRENT

257. MONITORING CHILDREN FOR THE DETECTION OF RECURRENT BACTERIURIA HAS BEEN ASSOCIATED WITH ALL OF THE FOLLOWING, EXCEPT:

A. Monitoring for recurrent bacteriuria by parents with a miniature qualitative culture (Testuria) has been unsuccessful
B. Incubation of sterile urine does not reduce the glucose concentration
C. Significant bacteriuria decreases urinary glucose concentrations to subnormal levels (less than 2 mg per 100 ml in morning fasting specimens)
D. A sensitive strip paper which is capable of reacting with small amounts of glucose normally present in the urine (Uriglox, KABI Labs) will distinguish significant bacteriuria from contamination
E. The strip test paper will not detect bacteriuria caused by pseudomonas aeruginosa

Ref. J Pediatr 78:851 1971
Ref. J Pediatr 78:859, 1971

CREATININE CLEARANCE

258. MOST CLINICAL CENTERS USE THE CLEARANCE OF ENDOGENOUS CREATININE AS THE STANDARD DETERMINANT OF RENAL FUNCTION. MANY TECHNICAL PROBLEMS CONTRIBUTE TO THE ACCURATE PERFORMANCE OF THE CREATININE CLEARANCE TEST IN CHILDREN. EACH OF THE FOLLOWING STATEMENTS IS CORRECT, EXCEPT:

A. A 24 hour urine collection makes the estimate of creatinine clearance more reliable
B. Accurate timing of each urine collection is important
C. Complete urine collections are necessary for accurate clearance values
D. The low plasma creatinine levels found in children with good renal function are difficult to measure
E. There are normal daily variations in creatinine clearance

Ref. Curr Probs in Pediatr 1:6, December, 1970

CYSTIC DISEASE OF KIDNEYS

259. THE MOST COMMON CYSTIC RENAL DISORDER IN CHILDHOOD IS:

A. Unilateral cystic dysplasia
B. Adult polycystic disease of kidneys and liver
C. Infantile polycystic disease
D. Cortical cysts with syndromes of multiple malformations (Down's, autosomal trisomies)
E. Medullary cystic disease

Ref. J Med Genetics 8:257, September, 1971

DIAGNOSTIC PROBLEM

260. A NINE MONTH- OLD INFANT WAS ADMITTED WITH A HISTORY OF FEVER AND DIARRHEA OF TWO DAYS DURATION. THE STOOLS HAVE BEEN BLOOD-TINGED, AND THE CHILD HAS HAD A TEN MINUTE GENERALIZED SEIZURE. NO URINE HAS BEEN PASSED FOR 12 HOURS.
PHYSICAL EXAMINATION REVEALS A BLOOD PRESSURE IN THE LEFT ARM OF 140/100 AND A FEW PETECHIAE ARE FOUND ON THE ANTERIOR CHEST. THE BUN IS 38, THE HEMOGLOBIN IS 6.5 GMS AND THE PLATELETS NUMBER 35,000. EXAMINATION OF THE BLOOD SMEAR REVEALS NUMEROUS FRAGMENTED AND DISTORTED ERYTHROCYTES. THE MOST LIKELY DIAGNOSIS IS:
A. Hemolytic-uremic syndrome
B. Acute glomerulonephritis
C. Acute salmonellosis
D. Meningococcemia
E. Systemic lupus erythematosus

Ref. Lancet
1:1123, June 7, 1969

ESTIMATION OF KIDNEY SIZE

261. THE AVERAGE KIDNEY LENGTH CORRESPONDS CLOSELY TO THE LENGTH OF THE FIRST FOUR LUMBAR VERTEBRAL BODIES THROUGHOUT CHILDHOOD, WITH THE EXCEPTION OF THE FIRST 1-1 1/2 YR. OF LIFE WHEN THE LENGTH OF THE NORMAL KIDNEY IS GREATER THAN THAT OF THIS SEGMENT OF THE SPINE. INCREASED SIZE OF THE KIDNEYS IN CHILDREN IS SEEN IN ALL OF THE FOLLOWING STATES, EXCEPT:
A. Beckwith's syndrome
B. Leukemia
C. Tyrosinosis
D. Neurolipidoses
E. Acute glomerulonephritis

Ref. Am J Roentgenol Radium
Ther Nucl Med
93:464, February, 1965

GLOMERULONEPHRITIS AND STREPTOCOCCI

262. IN A STUDY OF AN EPIDEMIC OF ACUTE DIFFUSE GLOMERULONEPHRITIS IN ISRAEL, ALL OF THE FOLLOWING OBSERVATIONS WERE CONFIRMED, EXCEPT:
A. The value of early antibiotic treatment of streptococcal infections in the prevention of rheumatic fever, is well recognized
B. The effectiveness of antimicrobial therapy in preventing acute glomerulonephritis in streptococcal pyodermas has not been proven
C. The incidence of acute glomerulonephritis following streptococcal pharyngitis is not altered by antibiotic therapy
D. The severity of acute glomerulonephritis which complicates streptococcal infections in children appears to be lessened by antibiotics
E. Eradication of the streptococcus by antibiotics does not influence the clinical course and duration of acute glomerulonephritis

Ref. J Infect Dis
124:141, August, 1971

HEMOLYTIC-UREMIC SYNDROME

263. THE HEMOLYTIC-UREMIC SYNDROME AFFECTS CHILDREN WHO ARE USUALLY LESS THAN ONE YEAR OF AGE, AND THE MOST COMMON ANTECEDENT EVENT IS:
A. Gastroenteritis,which is often bloody
B. Upper respiratory tract infection
C. Recent immunization with live attenuated virus
D. Bacteriuria
E. Pyoderma

Ref. J Pediatr 80:1, January 1972

HYPERKALEMIA

264. THE HIGHEST PRIORITY IN THE TREATMENT OF HYPERKALEMIA AND ACUTE RENAL FAILURE INVOLVES THE USE OF:
A. Intravenous 10% calcium gluconate
B. Sodium bicarbonate
C. 50% glucose and insulin
D. A sodium-potassium exchange resin
E. Peritoneal dialysis

Ref. Pediatrics 48:286, 1971

HYPERTENSION

265. A LOWERING OF ARTERIAL BLOOD PRESSURE IN HYPERTENSIVE EMERGENCIES MAY BE ACCOMPLISHED WITH REASONABLE SAFETY WITHIN A FEW SECONDS BY THE USE OF:
A. Reserpine
B. Hydralazine
C. Guanethidine
D. Intravenous diazoxide
E. Chlorothiazide

Ref. Pediatr Clin North Am 18:577, May, 1971

HYPOSPADIAS

266. HYPOSPADIAS SHOULD ALERT THE PEDIATRICIAN TO THE POSSIBILITY OF INTERSEX PROBLEMS. EACH OF THE FOLLOWING IS CORRECT, EXCEPT:
A. The presence of glandular or penile hypospadias in babies with both testes in the scrotum merits no further investigation of the patient's sex
B. In penoscrotal, scrotal, or perineal hypospadius sex determination is mandatory whether or not the testes are palpable in the scrotum
C. A family history may reveal hereditary forms of hypospadias
D. Elevated urinary excretion of 17-ketosteroids and pregnantriol confirms the diagnosis of maternal progestin treatment or congenital virilizing adrenal hyperplasia
E. If no testes are palpable in the scrotum in a newborn infant with hypospadias, and if the cells from buccal smears are sex chromatin positive, it is highly probable that the infant is a female pseudohermaphrodite

Ref. Acta Med Scand Supplement 203, 1970

NEPHRITIS, HENOCH-SCHONLEIN

267. THE NEPHRITIS OF HENOCH-SCHONLEIN PURPURA HAS BEEN ASSOCIATED WITH ALL OF THE FOLLOWING, EXCEPT:
A. Progression from focal to diffuse involvement
B. Mesangial deposits containing IgA, complement, fibrinogen and IgG
C. Normal serum complement levels
D. Minimal basement membrane involvement
E. Tendency for hematuria to recur

Ref. Pediatr Clin North Am 18:467, May, 1971

PROTEINURIA

268. FALSE POSITIVE TESTS FOR URINARY PROTEIN MAY RESULT FROM EACH OF THE FOLLOWING SUBSTANCES IN THE URINE, EXCEPT:
A. Radiologic contrast media
B. Zephiran
C. Penicillin
D. Sulfonamides
E. Tetracycline

Ref. Curr Probs in Pediatr 1:38, December, 1970

269. THE MOST COMMON CAUSE FOR MASSIVE PROTEINURIA IN CHILDREN IS:
A. A decreased tubular reabsorption of protein
B. An increased level in the plasma of one of the plasma proteins
C. Glomerular diseases
D. The presence of an abnormal protein in the plasma
E. An increased addition to the urine of tissue proteins from the genitourinary tract

Ref. Curr Probs in Pediatr 1:32, December, 1970

270. CHILDREN WITH PERSISTENT ORTHOSTATIC PROTEINURIA AND THOSE SPILLING MORE THAN 500 MGM OF PROTEIN PER DAY SHOULD BE SUBJECTED TO A RENAL BIOPSY. EACH OF THE FOLLOWING IS CORRECT, EXCEPT:
A. Orthostatic proteinuria is not a transient condition although data suggest an excellent 5-year prognosis
B. A decrease in protein excretion when a child assumes a recumbent position excludes renal disease
C. About half of children with fixed orthostatic proteinuria (present consistently in only the upright samples) have renal abnormalities by electron microscopy
D. Normal urine contains small quantities of protein
E. Proteinuria which is unrelated to posture is associated often with biopsy evidence of chronic glomerulonephritis

Ref. Curr Probs in Pediatr 1:41, December, 1970

RENAL TUBULAR ACIDOSIS

271. ONLY THE KIDNEY CAN REGULATE HYDROGEN ION BALANCE BY CONTROLLING THE CONCENTRATION OF BICARBONATE IN PLASMA. IN PRIMARY PROXIMAL RENAL TUBULAR ACIDOSIS ALL OF THE FOLLOWING ARE CORRECT, EXCEPT:

A. The patients exhibit hyperchloremic acidosis due to an isolated defect in bicarbonate reabsorption
B. All patients have been males
C. The only clinical manifestation is retarded growth
D. Children with proximal renal tubular acidosis can excrete a urine of strongly acid pH
E. The prognosis for growth recovery and spontaneous improvement is poor

Ref. Pediatr Clin North Am 18:535, May, 1971

272. SECONDARY PROXIMAL RENAL TUBULAR ACIDOSIS HAS BEEN ASSOCIATED WITH ALL OF THE FOLLOWING, EXCEPT:

A. Idiopathic Fanconi syndrome
B. Lowe's syndrome
C. Hyperglobulinemic states (sarcoid, active chronic hepatitis, Sjögren syndrome, etc.)
D. Wilson's disease
E. Outdated tetracycline

Ref. Pediatr Clin North Am 18:537, May, 1971

273. IN PRIMARY DISTAL RENAL TUBULAR ACIDOSIS ALL OF THE FOLLOWING ARE SEEN, EXCEPT:

A. The primary effect is an inability to establish adequate gradients of hydrogen ion between blood and tubular fluid
B. An inability to lower urinary pH below 6.0 is the most characteristic feature
C. The majority of cases are sporadic but several families have been reported in which the inheritance appears to be autosomal dominant with a variable degree of expression and greater penetrance in females
D. Nephrocalcinosis and secondary renal damage complicate inadequately-treated patients
E. The abnormality in primary distal renal tubular acidosis is transient

Ref. Pediatr Clin North Am 18:537, May, 1971

RENAL TUBULAR ACIDOSIS

274. SECONDARY DISTAL RENAL TUBULAR ACIDOSIS MAY BE ASSOCIATED WITH A NUMBER OF SYSTEMIC OR RENAL CONDITIONS INCLUDING EACH OF THE FOLLOWING, EXCEPT:

A. Vitamin D intoxication
B. Primary hyperparathyroidism
C. Renal homotransplantation
D. Lead poisoning
E. Amphotericin B nephropathy

Ref. Pediatr Clin North Am 18:540, May, 1971

275. THE DISTINCTION BETWEEN PROXIMAL AND DISTAL RENAL TUBULAR ACIDOSIS HAS IMPORTANT CLINICAL AS WELL AS THERAPEUTIC IMPLICATIONS. EACH OF THE FOLLOWING IS ACCEPTED AS CORRECT, <u>EXCEPT</u>:

A. Utilizing urinary pH, as the sole screening method in the detection of children with renal tubular acidosis, can no longer be considered adequate
B. The presence of an elevated urine pH at all levels of serum bicarbonate, despite the presence of severe systemic acidosis, characterizes distal renal tubular acidosis
C. The rate of calcium excretion in the urine is the most sensitive guide to therapy in distal renal tubular acidosis
D. As much as 10 mEq of citrate or bicarbonate per kg of body weight per day may be necessary to compensate for the large urinary loss of bicarbonate in proximal renal tubular acidosis
E. The administration of potassium is unnecessary in the therapy of distal renal tubular acidosis

Ref. Pediatr Clin North Am 18:541, May, 1971

SYPHILIS AND RENAL DISEASE

276. RENAL INVOLVEMENT IS AN UNCOMMON BUT WELL-DESCRIBED COMPLICATION OF SECONDARY SYPHILIS. EACH OF THE FOLLOWING IS A CLINICAL OR LABORATORY OBSERVATION OF THE KIDNEY DISEASE OF SYPHILIS, <u>EXCEPT</u>:

A. Identification of syphilitic antigen within the basement membrane
B. Spontaneous or therapy-induced remissions
C. A transient nephrotic syndrome
D. A clinical picture of acute glomerulonephritis
E. Deposition of immune complexes (IgG and complement) along the glomerular basement membrane

Ref. JAMA 216:1159, May 17, 1971

TRAUMA (URINARY TRACT)

277. HEMATURIA IS THE HALLMARK OF TRAUMATIC INJURY TO THE GENITOURINARY TRACT AND PROMPT INVESTIGATION IS ESSENTIAL. INTRAVENOUS PYELOGRAPHY IN CHILDREN WITH INJURIES TO THE GENITOURINARY TRACT WOULD BE LEAST LIKELY TO SHOW:

A. Unsuspected congenital abnormalities or tumor
B. Ureteral injury
C. Extravasation of opacified urine from the collecting system
D. Reduced amounts of contrast material within the urinary tract on the involved side
E. Bladder injury

Ref. Pediatr Digest 13:26, July, 1971

WORCESTERSHIRE SAUCE

278. A POTENTIALLY REVERSIBLE NEPHROPATHY HAS BEEN DESCRIBED IN ASSOCIATION WITH THE EXCESSIVE INTAKE OF WORCESTERSHIRE SAUCE WHICH HAS INCLUDED ALL OF THE FOLLOWING LABORATORY AND CLINICAL FEATURES, EXCEPT:

A. Hypertension
B. Generalized aminoaciduria
C. Renal calculi
D. Nephrotic syndrome
E. Urea nitrogen retention

Ref. Br Med J 3:6, July 3, 1971

FOR EACH OF THE FOLLOWING QUESTIONS, SELECT THE ONE APPROPRIATE ANSWER BY USING THE KEY OUTLINED BELOW:

1. If A, B and C are correct
2. If A and C are correct
3. If B and D are correct
4. If all are correct
5. If all are incorrect

ACUTE HEMORRHAGIC CYSTITIS

279. ACUTE HEMORRHAGIC CYSTITIS IS A NOT UNCOMMON DISEASE OF CHILDREN WHICH OFTEN PRESENTS A PROBLEM IN THE DIFFERENTIAL DIAGNOSIS OF HEMATURIA. WHICH OF THE FOLLOWING ORGANISMS HAVE BEEN RELATED TO THIS ENTITY?:

A. Mumps
B. Escherichia coli
C. Coxsackie viruses
D. Adenoviruses
E. Herpes simplex

Ref. Amer J Dis Child
121:281, April, 1971

AMPICILLIN AND URINE EXAMINATIONS

280. PRIOR TREATMENT OF CHILDREN WITH AMPICILLIN MAY LEAD TO CONFUSION IN WHICH OF THE FOLLOWING EXAMINATIONS OF URINE?:

A. False positive spots for leucine/isoleucine on amino acid chromatogram
B. False positive spot for phenylalanine in paper electrophoretograms
C. Crystalluria and an acid urine
D. Positive test for reducing substances
E. Positive test for urinary protein

Ref. Pediatrics
48:638, October, 1971

CYSTIC DISEASES OF THE LIVER AND KIDNEY

281. WHICH OF THE FOLLOWING GENETIC DISORDERS ARE ASSOCIATED WITH CYSTIC CHANGES IN THE KIDNEYS AND LIVER?:

A. Infantile polycystic disease of the kidneys
B. Meckel syndrome
C. Zellweger (Smith-Opitz-Inhorn) syndrome
D. Medullary sponge kidney disease
E. Congenital hepatic fibrosis

Ref. Paediatrica Universitatis Tokyo
18:112, December, 1970

DIURETICS

282. THE RISK OF IATROGENIC SIDE-EFFECTS OF DIURETIC THERAPY DEMANDS AN UNDERSTANDING OF UNDERLYING PATHOPHYSIOLOGIC MECHANISMS IN TREATING EDEMA IN CHILDREN TO AVOID WHICH OF THE FOLLOWING REACTIONS?:

A. Azotemia
B. Hyperuricemia
C. Hypokalemic alkalosis
D. Dilutional hyponatremia
E. Deafness

Ref. Pediatr Clin N Am
18:561, May, 1971

GLOMERULONEPHRITIS AND VIRUSES

283. CLINICAL GLOMERULONEPHRITIS HAS BEEN REPORTED IN HUMANS WITH WHICH OF THE FOLLOWING VIRAL ANTIGENS?:
A. Mumps
B. Measles
C. Vaccinia
D. Adenoviruses
E. Coxsackie and ECHO viruses

Ref. Pediatr Clin N Am 18:467, May, 1971

HEMODIALYSIS

284. EXTENDED HEMODIALYSIS IN CHILDREN HAS A STRESSFUL IMPACT ON PATIENTS, FAMILIES AND STAFF. OTHER COMPLICATIONS HAVE INCLUDED WHICH OF THE FOLLOWING?:
A. Shunt infections
B. Clotting episodes
C. Convulsions
D. Pericarditis
E. Peripheral neuropathy

Ref. Pediatr Clin N Amer 18:625, May, 1971

HEMOLYTIC-UREMIC SYNDROME

285. THE HEMOLYTIC-UREMIC SYNDROME OF INFANCY IS CHARACTERIZED BY WHICH OF THE FOLLOWING?:
A. No increase in patient survival with heparin therapy
B. 50 percent of survivors demonstrate chronic renal disease
C. Decreased platelet and red cell survival during acute phase
D. Sequestration of platelets in spleen rather than in microcirculation of kidneys by external counting and scintiscan
E. Rate of destruction of transfused platelets is less rapid than in immune thrombocytopenias

Ref. J Pediatr 78:426, 1971

HYPERKALEMIA

286. CHILDREN WITH SUSPECTED HYPERKALEMIA COMPLICATING ACUTE RENAL FAILURE MAY SHOW WHICH OF THE FOLLOWING ECG ABNORMALITIES?:
A. Prolonged QRS complexes
B. Depressed ST segment
C. High T wave
D. Heart block
E. Fibrillation

Ref. Pediatrics 48:286, 1971

KIDNEYS, DYSPLASIA

287. ABNORMAL DEVELOPMENT OF NEPHRONIC AND DUCTAL STRUCTURES WHICH RESULTS IN RENAL DYSPLASIA IS ALWAYS ASSOCIATED WITH WHICH OF THE FOLLOWING?:
A. Familial tendency
B. Dysplastic ducts
C. Cysts
D. Nests of metaplastic cartilage
E. Lower urinary tract obstruction

Ref. Pediatr Clin N Am 18:395, 1971

NEPHROTIC SYNDROME

288. AMONG THE DISEASES TO BE CONSIDERED IN THE DIFFERENTIAL DIAGNOSIS OF THE NEPHROTIC SYNDROME IN EARLY INFANCY ARE:

A. Congenital nephrosis (microcystic disease)
B. Idiopathic nephrotic syndrome (minimal lesion syndrome)
C. Renal vein thrombosis
D. Hereditary onycho-osteodysplasia
E. Congenital syphilis

Ref. Pediatrics 49:260, 1972

POLYCYSTIC DISEASE

289. INFANTILE POLYCYSTIC DISEASE MAY PRESENT BEYOND THE PERINATAL PERIOD WITH VARYING DEGREES OF SEVERITY AND MAY BE ASSOCIATED WITH WHICH OF THE FOLLOWING?:

A. Portal hypertension
B. Periportal hepatic fibrosis
C. Hepatomegaly
D. Dilated and infolded bile ducts
E. Progressive renal failure

Ref. J Med Genetics 8:257, September, 1971

290. INFANTILE POLYCYSTIC DISEASE MAY PRESENT IN THE NEWBORN WITH WHICH OF THE FOLLOWING ASSOCIATIONS?:

A. Potter's facies
B. Cysts which are fairly uniform in size and distributed throughout the cortex and medulla
C. Abdominal distention due to marked renal enlargement
D. Polyhydramnios
E. Dominant inheritance

Ref. Ped Clin N Am 18:435, May, 1971

THIRD FACTOR

291. THE EXPANSION OF THE EXTRACELLULAR FLUID COMPARTMENT DEPENDS ULTIMATELY ON SALT AND WATER RETENTION BY THE KIDNEYS. ALDOSTERONE AND GLOMERULAR FILTRATION RATES ARE RECOGNIZED AS HAVING A CONTROLLING INFLUENCE ON SALT BALANCE. OTHER PROPOSED MECHANISMS UNDER STUDY WHICH HAVE BEEN LABELED AS "THIRD FACTOR(S)" HAVE INVOLVED WHICH OF THE FOLLOWING?:

A. Intrarenal distribution of blood flow
B. Estrogens
C. Angiotensin
D. Prostaglandins
E. Kinins

Ref. Ped Clin N Am 18:561, May, 1971

TRANSPLANTATION, RENAL

292. CHRONIC HEMODIALYSIS AND RENAL TRANSPLANTATION HAVE BECOME FEASIBLE IN CERTAIN CHILDREN WITH VIRTUAL ABSENCE OF RENAL FUNCTION. WHICH OF THE FOLLOWING AID IN THE DIAGNOSIS OF HOMOGRAFT REJECTION?:

A. Decreasing urinary output
B. Increasing BUN
C. Diminishing creatinine clearance
D. Fever
E. Local tenderness

Ref. J Pediatr Surg 6:245, June, 1971

TURNER'S SYNDROME AND RENAL ANOMALIES

293. IN A STUDY OF RENAL ANOMALIES IN TURNER'S SYNDROME, WHICH OF THE FOLLOWING OBSERVATIONS WERE SUGGESTED IN THEIR EMBRYOGENESIS, INCIDENCE AND CLINICAL SIGNIFICANCE?:
A. The renal anomalies represent varying degrees of "failure of ascent and rotation" of the kidneys during fetal life
B. The horseshoe kidney is the most complete expression of a continuum of morphologic abnormalities
C. The majority of children have either horseshoe kidneys or low placement and malrotation
D. Most of the children had evidence of impaired renal function
E. Most of the patients have an abnormal urinalysis

Ref. Clin Pediatr
10:561, October, 1971

VESICOURETERAL REFLUX

294. IN A STUDY OF 115 CHILDREN WITH VESICOURETERAL REFLUX WHO HAD BEEN FOLLOWED FOR 5 OR MORE YEARS, WHICH OF THE FOLLOWING WERE SUGGESTED?:
A. Vesicoureteral reflux is found more often in girls
B. Reflux does not appear to be related to the rate of recurrence of bacteriuria in girls
C. The majority of the children studied had normal cystography
D. The necropsy incidence of chronic pyelonephritis is much higher in females
E. Reflux appears to initiate, propagate and accompany the radiographic findings ascribed to chronic pyelonephritis

Ref. Pediatrics
48:782, November, 1971

HYPERTENSION

MATCH THE DRUG WITH THE MOST FITTING AND COMMON SIDE-EFFECT WHICH MAY BE EXPERIENCED IN THE MEDICAL MANAGEMENT OF HYPERTENSION IN CHILDREN:

295. ___ Hyperkalemia
296. ___ Nasal congestion
297. ___ Lupus-like and arthritis syndromes
298. ___ Hyperuricemia
299. ___ Postural hypotension

A. Chlorothiazide
B. Hydralazine
C. Reserpine
D. Spironolactone
E. Guanethidine

Ref. Pediatr Clin N Am
18:577, May, 1971

EDEMA

MATCH THE MECHANISM WITH THE CLINICAL STATE WHICH RESULTS IN AN EXPANSION OF THE INTERSTITIAL COMPARTMENT AND EXPRESSION IN THE CHILD AS EDEMA:

300. ___ Protein-losing enteropathy
301. ___ Vitamin E deficiency
302. ___ Incompatible blood transfusion
303. ___ Cirrhosis
304. ___ Gonadal dysgenesis
305. ___ Angioneurotic edema

A. Capillary leak
B. Lymphatic obstruction
C. Hypoalbuminemia
D. Reduced glomerular filtration

Ref. Pediatr Clin N Am
18:561, May, 1971

FOR EACH OF THE FOLLOWING MULTIPLE CHOICE QUESTIONS, SELECT THE ONE MOST APPROPRIATE ANSWER:

CARDIAC FAILURE

306. NINETY PER CENT OF INFANTS WITH CONGENITAL HEART DISEASE WHO DEVELOP CONGESTIVE HEART FAILURE DO SO DURING THE FIRST YEAR OF LIFE. WHICH OF THE FOLLOWING IS LEAST LIKELY TO BE ASSOCIATED WITH FAILURE IN THE FIRST FEW MONTHS OF LIFE?:
A. Transposition of the great vessels
B. Large interventricular septal defect
C. Aortic atresia
D. Hypoplasia of the left ventricle
E. Atrial septal defect

Ref. Pediatrics 47:1057, June, 1971

307. AN INFANT WHO HAS DEVELOPED CONGESTIVE HEART FAILURE (COMBINED RIGHT AND LEFT VENTRICULAR FAILURE) IS LEAST LIKELY TO SHOW WHICH OF THE FOLLOWING SIGNS AND SYMPTOMS?:
A. Cardiomegaly
B. Hepatomegaly
C. Peripheral edema
D. Feeding difficulties with growth failure
E. Tachypnea during sleep

Ref. Pediatrics 47:1057, June, 1971

308. AN AGGRESSIVE APPROACH TO MEDICAL TREATMENT FOR AN INFANT WITH CONGESTIVE HEART FAILURE IS CRUCIAL IF A BABY IS TO BE SALVAGED BY SURGERY. THE MOST POPULAR GLYCOSIDE OF DIGITALIS FOR PEDIATRIC USE HAS BEEN DIGOXIN. WHICH OF THE FOLLOWING IS THE MOST IMPORTANT CLUE TO TOXICITY IN THE USE OF DIGOXIN IN INFANTS?:
A. Serum electrolytes
B. Electrocardiographic monitoring
C. Vomiting
D. Diarrhea
E. Anorexia

Ref. Pediatrics 47:1060, June, 1971

309. AN INFANT IN CONGESTIVE HEART FAILURE WHO PRESENTS EITHER WITH IMPENDING OR OVERT PULMONARY EDEMA IS LEAST LIKELY TO BE HELPED THERAPEUTICALLY BY WHICH OF THE FOLLOWING?:
A. Morphine sulfate
B. Ethacrynic acid
C. Oxygen
D. Recumbent positioning
E. Digoxin

Ref. Pediatrics 47:1060, June, 1971

CIRCULATORY CHANGES AT BIRTH

310. THE PRINCIPAL CIRCULATORY CHANGES THAT OCCUR AT BIRTH INVOLVE ALL OF THE FOLLOWING, EXCEPT:
A. Spectacular fall in pulmonary vascular resistance
B. Rise in systemic vascular resistance
C. Increase in blood flow to the right atrium associated with abolition of umbilical venous return
D. Increase in flow to the left atrium via the expanded lungs
E. Constriction of the patient ductus arteriosus in response to a rise in systemic arterial pO_2

Ref. Pediatr Portfolio 1:No 13, March 21, 1971

CONGENITAL HEART DISEASE

311. AN X-RAY OF THE CHEST IN A CHILD WITH A LARGE INTERATRIAL SEPTAL DEFECT WOULD BE LIKELY TO SHOW ALL OF THE FOLLOWING, EXCEPT:
A. A large pulmonary artery
B. Right ventricular enlargement
C. Increased pulmonary vasculature
D. Right atrial enlargement
E. Left atrial enlargement

Ref. Pediatr Clin N Am 17:967, November, 1970

ENDOCARDIAL FIBROELASTOSIS

312. ENDOCARDIAL FIBROELASTOSIS IS PROBABLY OVERDIAGNOSED MORE OFTEN THAN IT IS MISSED BY PEDIATRICIANS. HOWEVER, ALL OF THE FOLLOWING STATEMENTS ARE CORRECT, EXCEPT:
A. Cardiac decompensation with rapid onset in a previously well child is a characteristic feature
B. Symptoms usually begin after the first month of life
C. Mitral regurgitation is clinically recognizable in about one-half of the children
D. The electrocardiogram shows a pattern of extreme left ventricular hypertrophy with T-wave flattening or inversion in the left precordial leads of most children
E. Endocardial fibroelastosis is not observed with other malformations of the heart and great vessels

Ref. Clin. Pediatr 10:246, May, 1971

313. HYPERTENSION, HYPOSTHENURIA AND NITROGEN RETENTION DEVELOPING IN A CHILD WITH SEVERE BURNS AFTER PROLONGED IMMOBLIZATION MAY BE ACCOMPANIED BY AN INCREASE IN SERUM:
A. Calcium
B. Phosphorus
C. Potassium
D. Sodium
E. Magnesium

Ref. Pediatrics 49:92, 1972

DIAGNOSTIC PROBLEM

314. A 16 WEEK-OLD INFANT WITH AN URTICARIAL RASH, FEVER, CONJUNCTIVITIS AND AN ELECTROCARDIOGRAM SUGGESTIVE OF MYOCARDIAL INFARCTION SHOULD BE SUSPECTED OF HAVING:
A. Infantile polyarteritis nodosa
B. Systemic lupus erythematosus
C. Takayasu's disease
D. Giant cell arteritis
E. Rheumatic carditis with necrotizing angiitis of the coronary arteries

Ref. J Pediatr 78:1039, June, 1971

RHEUMATOID ARTHRITIS

315. THE ACUTE FEBRILE ONSET OF JUVENILE RHEUMATOID ARTHRITIS REPRESENTS ONE OF THE MOST COMMON FEVERS OF UNKNOWN ORIGIN WHICH IS REFERRED TO A CHILDREN'S HOSPITAL. EACH OF THE FOLLOWING REGARDING CLASSIC STILL'S DISEASE IS CORRECT, EXCEPT:

A. The children often lack articular manifestations other than arthralgia
B. Large diurnal deflections in fever are characteristic with one or two daily peaks
C. A migratory macular salmon-pink rash may occur on the trunk, neck and extremities which is virtually pathognomonic
D. These children are at significant risk of developing iridocyclitis
E. Generalized lymphadenopathy is common

Ref. J Pediatr
77:355, September, 1970

RHEUMATOID ARTHRITIS AND THE LIVER

316. THE HEPATIC INVOLVEMENT WHICH MAY BE SEEN IN THE COURSE OF JUVENILE RHEUMATOID ARTHRITIS MAY BE ASSOCIATED WITH ALL OF THE FOLLOWING, EXCEPT:

A. Active, often severe, and usually the febrile systemic form of rheumatoid arthritis
B. Mild and nonprogressive liver disease
C. Marked degree of hepatomegaly
D. Severe hepatic dysfunction which may occasionally lead to chronic liver disease
E. Minor abnormalities in liver function studies such as transaminase activities, bilirubin and bromsulphalein retention

Ref. J Pediatr
79:139, July, 1971

317. THE OBSERVATION THAT RHEUMATOID ARTHRITIS MAY REMIT TEMPORARILY IN PATIENTS WHO CONTRACT INTERCURRENT LIVER DISEASE WAS NOTED BY STILL IN HIS CLASSIC DESCRIPTION OF JUVENILE RHEUMATOID ARTHRITIS IN 1897. THIS PHENOMENON HAS BEEN OBSERVED IN ALL OF THE FOLLOWING ENTITIES, EXCEPT:

A. Infectious hepatitis
B. Drug induced hepatitis
C. Biliary obstruction
D. Pregnancy
E. Chronic active hepatitis or plasma cell hepatitis

Ref. J Pediatr
79:139, July, 1971

RHEUMATIC FEVER, ACUTE PHASE REACTANTS

318. TESTS WHICH MAY DETECT AN INFLAMMATORY STATE ARE OF VALUE IN THE LABORATORY DIAGNOSIS OF CHILDREN WITH POSSIBLE RHEUMATIC FEVER. ALL OF THE FOLLOWING ARE TRUE, EXCEPT:

A. The erythrocyte sedimentation rate in patients with rheumatic carditis complicated by heart failure is usually normal
B. Persistent elevation of the erythrocyte sedimentation rate does not imply a poor prognosis in rheumatic fever
C. Persistence or reappearance of a positive C-reactive protein often suggests a "chronic" attack of rheumatic fever
D. Elevation of the erythrocyte sedimentation rate and the C-reactive protein may be related to injections of benzathine penicillin
E. A normal erythrocyte sedimentation rate and a negative C-reactive protein should cast doubt on the diagnosis of rheumatic fever

Ref. Pediatr Clin N Am
18:138, February, 1971

TACHYCARDIA, SUPRAVENTRICULAR

319. EXCLUDING THE WOLFF-PARKINSON-WHITE SYNDROME, CONGENITAL AND ACQUIRED HEART DISEASE, AND POSTOPERATIVE ARRHYTHMIAS, PAROXYSMAL ATRIAL TACHYCARDIA CAN BE CLASSIFIED INTO TWO SEPARATE GROUPS WHICH ARE AGE-RELATED. EACH OF THE FOLLOWING IS CHARACTERISTIC OF P.A.T., EXCEPT:

A. The disease appears to be self-limiting in infants
B. The diagnosis in infants is not made frequently until after the development of congestive heart failure
C. About one-half of infants have but a single attack
D. Digoxin, quinidine and propranolol have a striking ability to prevent recurrences in older children
E. Under the age of four months most of the infants with P. A. T. are males

Ref. Lancet
p.832, April 24, 1971

TACHYCARDIA, SUPRAVENTRICULAR

320. IN INFANTS AND CHILDREN SUPRAVENTRICULAR TACHYCARDIA WOULD BE LEAST LIKELY TO BE ASSOCIATED WITH:

A. Normal hearts
B. Cardiomyopathies
C. Ebstein's anomaly
D. Cyanotic syncopal attacks (cerebrovascular insufficiency) in tetralogy of Fallot
E. Wolff-Parkinson-White syndrome

Ref. N Engl J Med
284:1359, June 17, 1971

UMBILICAL VESSEL CATHETERIZATION

321. CLINICAL AND AUTOPSY COMPLICATION RATES IN THE USE OF UMBILICAL VESSEL CATHETERS IN MANY SERIES APPEARS IN THE ORDER OF 10 PER CENT. THE MOST COMMON AND MOST SEVERE COMPLICATION HAS BEEN:

A. Infection
B. Cardiac arrhythmias
C. Hemorrhage
D. Thrombosis and hemorrhagic infarction
E. Placement of catheters outside the vascular system

Ref. Amer J Dis Child
121:213, March, 1971

VASCULAR ANOMALIES

322. THE CLINICAL PATTERNS OF ANOMALIES OF THE AORTIC ARCH ARE EXTREMELY VARIABLE. EACH OF THE FOLLOWING IS CORRECT, EXCEPT:

A. A "pulmonary sling" refers to an anomalous left pulmonary artery arising from the main trunk to the right of the midline causing anterior displacement and narrowing of the right main stem bronchus
B. An anomalous retro-esophageal subclavian artery seldom produces dysphagia
C. A simple right aortic arch produces no symptoms
D. A right aortic arch is rarely associated with other anomalies of the heart
E. A ring around the trachea and esophagus may be formed by a right arch and ligamentum arteriosum

Ref. Mayo Clin Proc
46:182, March, 1971

VASCULAR RINGS, DOUBLE AORTIC ARCH

323. MALFORMATIONS OF THE AORTIC ARCH SYSTEM MAY, BY COMPRESSION OF THE TRACHEA AND ESOPHAGUS, CAUSE RESPIRATORY DISTRESS AND DYSPHAGIA. EACH OF THE FOLLOWING IS CORRECT IN REGARD TO A DOUBLE AORTIC ARCH, EXCEPT:

A. When the vascular ring is not tight there may be no symptoms
B. A double aortic arch is rarely associated with other anomalies of the heart
C. A wheezy type of respiration that is heard when the child is awake or asleep is a common clinical observation
D. Flexion of the neck usually increases the respiratory difficulty
E. Surgical correction results in immediate disappearance of symptoms in all babies

Ref. Mayo Clin Proc
46:183, March, 1971

FOR EACH OF THE FOLLOWING QUESTIONS, SELECT THE ONE APPROPRIATE ANSWER BY USING THE KEY OUTLINED BELOW:

1. If A, B and C are correct
2. If A and C are correct
3. If B and D are correct
4. If all are correct
5. If all are incorrect

CARDIAC ARRHYTHMIAS

324. BRADYCARDIA AND APNEA HAVE BEEN ASSOCIATED WITH WHICH OF THE FOLLOWING?:

A. Transtracheal aspiration
B. Nasopharyngeal suctioning of newborn
C. Gavage feedings
D. Insertion of endotracheal tube
E. Introduction of bronchoscope

Ref. J Pediatr
78:441, March, 1971

CARDIAC CATHETERIZATION AND FEVER

325. FEBRILE EPISODES FOLLOWING CARDIAC CATHETERIZATION AND ANGIOGRAPHY OCCUR IN ABOUT ONE-THIRD OF CHILDREN. WHICH OF THE FOLLOWING STATEMENTS ARE CORRECT?:

A. Blood cultures from sites other than the catheter are commonly positive during cardiac catheterization
B. Elevated temperatures following cardiac catheterization return to normal in most children within 24 hours
C. Antibiotic prophylaxis prevents most febrile reactions
D. Fever is related to the number of injections of contrast material
E. Fever is related to the duration and extent of the manipulation

Ref. J Pediatr
80:215, February, 1972

TETRALOGY OF FALLOT - OPERATIVE COMPLICATIONS

326. THE MAJOR LONG RANGE COMPLICATION OF AORTOPULMONARY ANASTOMOSIS FOR TETRALOGY OF FALLOT IS RELATED TO EXCESSIVELY LARGE OPERATIVE SHUNTS.
THE RECOGNITION OF A LARGE LEFT-TO-RIGHT SHUNT THROUGH THE ANASTOMOSIS SHOULD BE ENHANCED BY WHICH OF THE FOLLOWING?:

A. Almost complete absence of cyanosis following anastomosis
B. A short, low-pitched rough continuous murmer postoperatively
C. Progressive prominence of the pulmonary artery segment
D. Marked increase in pulmonary vascular markings
E. Combined ventricular hypertrophy

Ref. Circulation
43:263, 1971

CONGENITAL HEART DISEASE

IN THE RADIOLOGICAL EXAMINATION OF THE CHILD WITH CONGENITAL HEART DISEASE AN APPROPRIATE DIAGNOSIS MAY BE SUGGESTED BY A CAREFUL INTERPRETATION OF THE INTRAPULMONARY VASCULATURE AS WELL AS THE SIZE AND CONFIGURATION OF THE HEART:

MATCH THE FOLLOWING:

327. ___ Transposition of great vessels with pulmonary stenosis
328. ___ Coarctation of aorta
329. ___ Small shunt (less than 2:1)
330. ___ Endocardial fibroelastosis

A. Pulmonary vasculature normal
B. Cardiac enlargement
C. Both
D. Neither

Ref. The Roentgen Diagnosis of Congenital Heart Disease
Congenital Heart Disease
Vol. 2, No. 1, Page 117
Cardiovascular Clinics

MATCH THE FOLLOWING:

331. ___ Tetralogy of Fallot
332. ___ Tricuspid atresia
333. ___ Pulmonary stenosis
334. ___ Ebstein's anomaly

A. Pulmonary vasculature decreased
B. Cardiac enlargement
C. Both
D. Neither

Ref. The Roentgen Diagnosis of Congenital Heart Disease
Congenital Heart Disease
Vol. 2, No. 1, Page 121
Cardiovascular Clinics

MATCH THE FOLLOWING:

335. ___ Hypoplastic left heart syndrome
336. ___ Mitral insufficiency (primary)
337. ___ Obstructive anomalous pulmonary venous return
338. ___ Aortic stenosis

A. Pulmonary vasculature congested
B. Cardiac enlargement
C. Both
D. Neither

Ref. The Roentgen Diagnosis of Congenital Heart Disease
Congenital Heart Disease
Vol. 2, No. 1, Page 132
Cardiovascular Clinics

HYPERTENSION

EVERY CHILD WITH PERSISTENT, UNEXPLAINED DIASTOLIC HYPERTENSION DESERVES A THOROUGH DIAGNOSTIC STUDY. MATCH THE CAUSES FOR HYPERTENSION WITH THE APPROPRIATE LABORATORY TESTS WHICH MIGHT SUGGEST THE DIAGNOSIS. MORE THAN ONE ANSWER MAY APPLY:

339. ___ Cushing's disease
340. ___ Renovascular hypertension
341. ___ Acute post-streptococcal glomerulonephritis
342. ___ Systemic lupus erythematosus
343. ___ Familial dysautonomia
344. ___ Pheochromocytoma
345. ___ Neuroblastoma
346. ___ Adrenogenital syndrome
347. ___ Unilateral renal parenchymal disease
348. ___ Aldosteronism

A. 24 hr urine for VMA and HVA
B. 24 hr urine for 17- hydroxysteroids and 17- ketosteroids
C. Immunoelectrophoresis
D. Two hour postprandial blood sugar
E. Fast-sequence intravenous pyelogram
F. CO_2, Cl, Na, K, BUN, creatinine

Ref. Pediatr Clin N Am
18:1283, November, 1971

FOR EACH OF THE FOLLOWING MULTIPLE CHOICE QUESTIONS, SELECT THE ONE APPROPRIATE ANSWER:

MYCOPLASMA, T-STRAINS

349. T-STAINS OF MYCOPLASMA HAVE HAD AN ASSOCIATION WITH ALL OF THE FOLLOWING, EXCEPT:
A. Congenital malformations
B. Bronchopneumonic lungs in an aborted fetus
C. Premature deliveries with accompanying maternal febrile illness
D. Isolation from chorion, decidua and amnion and spontaneous abortion
E. Recovery from the male and female human urogenital tracts

Ref. N Engl J Med
285:950, October 21, 1971

AMPICILLIN AND BODY RASHES

350. WHEN A CHILD IS BEING TREATED WITH AMPICILLIN AND HE DEVELOPS A GENERALIZED MACULOPAPULAR RASH, THE PHYSICIAN SHOULD CONSIDER IN HIS DIFFERENTIAL DIAGNOSIS:
A. 6-amino-penicillanic acid hypersensitivity
B. Erythema multiforme
C. Infectious mononucleosis
D. Enteroviral exanthem
E. Streptococcal exanthem

Ref. Clin Pediatr
10:59, January, 1971

AMPICILLIN, SODIUM AND STABILITY

351. ANTIBIOTIC STABILITY IN PARENTERAL SOLUTIONS IS CRITICAL IF FULL THERAPEUTIC EFFECTIVENESS IS TO BE OBTAINED. SODIUM AMPICILLIN IS RAPIDLY INACTIVATED IN ALL OF THE FOLLOWING SOLUTIONS, EXCEPT:
A. Lactated Ringer's
B. Dextrose 5% in water
C. Dextrose 10% in water
D. Dextrose 5% in normal saline
E. Electrolyte solutions containing acetate rather than lactate

Ref. Pediatrics
49:22, January, 1972

AUSTRALIA ANTIGEN

352. BLOOD TRANSFUSIONS IN THE UNITED STATES HAVE BEEN ESTIMATED TO CAUSE AN ANNUAL INCIDENCE OF 30,000 CASES OF HEPATITIS, WITH JAUNDICE, 150,000 CASES OF ANICTERIC HEPATITIS, AND 3,000 DEATHS. ALL OF THE FOLLOWING ARE CORRECT IN REGARD TO SERUM HEPATITIS, EXCEPT:
A. The virus of serum hepatitis (virus B) like the virus of infectious hepatitis (virus A) is transmissible by mouth as well as by injection
B. The Australia antigen (hepatitis-associated antigen) is transient in most patients with icteric serum hepatitis
C. The Australia antigen is more prone to persist for a long period of time in patients with anicteric serum hepatitis
D. A negative test for Australia antigen rules out the possibility of transmitting serum hepatitis by blood transfusion
E. There has been a curious association of the Australia antigen in children with leukemia, Hodgkin's disease and Down's syndrome

Ref. J Pediatr
78:887, May, 1971

CAT-SCRATCH DISEASE

353. CAT-SCRATCH DISEASE IS ONE OF THE MOST COMMON CAUSES OF REGIONAL ADENITIS AND IS OFTEN UNRECOGNIZED BECAUSE OF THE MILD CLINICAL COURSE WHICH IS FREQUENTLY SEEN.
EACH OF THE FOLLOWING IS CORRECT IN CAT-SCRATCH DISEASE, EXCEPT:

A. Eosinophilia is a constant laboratory finding
B. An inoculation site can be found as long as two to three months after contact in some cases
C. Suppuration of lymph nodes occurs in only about 10 per cent of cases
D. The skin test is positive in nearly 100 per cent of cases
E. Nearly all patients have had a history of contact with cats

Ref. JAMA
207:312, January 13, 1969

CHOLERA

354. IN 1970, CHOLERA SPREAD WESTWARD FROM THE INDIAN SUB-CONTINENT INTO EASTERN EUROPE AND INTO NORTH AND WEST AFRICA. THE EL TOR VIBRIO REPLACED THE "CLASSICAL" CHOLERA VIBRIO EXCEPT IN EAST PAKISTAN. CHOLERA DUE TO THE EL TOR VIBRIO DIFFERS FROM CLASSICAL V. CHOLERAE IN ALL OF THE FOLLOWING RESPECTS, EXCEPT:

A. Vaccination is an efficient method of preventing the spread of cholera
B. Mild and asymptomatic cases appear to occur more frequently with El Tor infection
C. Chronic carriers of the El Tor biotype have been observed
D. The El Tor vibrio is more resistant and survives longer in the environment
E. The El Tor vibrio causes fewer secondary cases in affected families

Ref. Clin Pediatr
10:483, August, 1971

CONGENITAL SYPHILIS

355. THE DECISION TO TREAT A CHILD WHO IS NORMAL CLINICALLY BUT WHO HAS A POSITIVE SEROLOGIC TEST FOR SYPHILIS IS A DIFFICULT ONE TO MAKE FOR A PHYSICIAN. EACH OF THE FOLLOWING STATEMENTS IN REGARD TO CONGENITAL SYPHILIS IS CORRECT, EXCEPT:

A. Severe congenital syphilis has been reported without detectable levels of fetal IgM
B. An infant may not develop clinical syphilis for one to two months after birth when the maternal disease has been acquired late in pregnancy
C. A mother who acquires syphilis late in pregnancy may give birth to an infant with a negative serologic test for syphilis, especially if a flocculation rather than a complement-fixation test is employed
D. The titer of passively transferred VDRL (Venereal Disease Research Laboratory) antibody in the infant is consistently lower than the antibody titer in the mother's serum
E. The passively transferred antibody in the infant declines sharply in the first two months or three months of life in the absence of infection in the child

Ref. N Engl J Med
284:642, March 25, 1971

CYTOMEGALOVIRUS INFECTIONS

356. IT HAS BEEN KNOWN FOR MANY YEARS THAT CYTOMEGALOVIRUS (CMV) CAN INDUCE PROFOUND BRAIN DAMAGE IN THE FETUS. SCREENING OF NEWBORN INFANT POPULATIONS HAS LED TO ALL OF THE FOLLOWING OBSERVATIONS IN CONGENITAL CMV INFECTIONS, EXCEPT:

A. CMV has been found in the urine of approximately 6 to 15 of 1,000 live births in multiple surveys
B. Isolation of the virus is the most sensitive means of detecting CMV infections in newborn infants
C. 19S CMV-specific macroglobulin may persist in the infant into the second year of life and perhaps longer
D. All newborns with 19S immunofluorescent antibody to CMV in their sera appear to be symptomatic
E. Viruria is not uncommon in the absence of CMV-specific macroglobulin in the cord blood of infants

Ref. J Infect Dis
123:555, May, 1971

357. VIRURIA IN CONGENITAL CYTOMEGALOVIRUS (CMV) INFECTIONS HAS BEEN SHOWN TO PERSIST FOR AS LONG AS EIGHT YEARS. ALL OF THE FOLLOWING IMMUNOLOGICAL OBSERVATIONS HAVE BEEN MADE IN THIS DISEASE, EXCEPT:

A. Evidence exists that the presence of maternal antibody alone is sufficient to protect the fetus from infection
B. Infected infants are capable of forming neutralizing and complement-fixing antibody
C. Lymphocytes from infected infants respond normally to phytohemagglutinin stimulation
D. Infants infected with CMV are able to produce interferon
E. CMV has been demonstrated in the lymphocytes of congenitally infected infants for several months after birth

Ref. J Infect Dis
123:555, May, 1971

CYTOMEGALOVIRUS DISEASE

358. IN BABIES WITH INTRAUTERINE CYTOMEGALOVIRUS INFECTION ALL OF THE FOLLOWING HAVE BEEN OBSERVED, EXCEPT:

A. Placental infection without fetal involvement has been demonstrated following primary cytomegalovirus infection during pregnancy
B. The critical period during pregnancy when maternal infection carries a risk for the fetus is unknown
C. Complement-fixing antibody titers can fall during the first few months of life in congenitally infected infants
D. The absence of inclusion bodies in sections of the placenta does not exclude the presence of cytomegalovirus
E. The titer of virus in the urine of infected infants is considerably lower than that in the urine of infected adults

Ref. J Pediatr
79:401, September, 1971

CYTOMEGALOVIRUS

359. CYTOMEGALOVIRUSES APPEAR TO BE ENDEMIC IN ALL HUMAN SOCIETIES, AND THE GREAT MAJORITY OF INFECTED BABIES ARE ASYMPTOMATIC. EACH OF THE FOLLOWING IS CORRECT IN REGARD TO INFECTION WITH CYTOMEGALOVIRUSES, EXCEPT:

A. In the United States infection is acquired at an earlier age by children of low economic status
B. There is usually no history of maternal illness that might assist in the timing of the infection of the fetus
C. A congenitally infected infant is often the first born to a young woman
D. No evidence exists that a woman may give birth to a second congenitally infected and damaged infant
E. Intra-uterine transfusion with fresh blood may induce fetal infection

Ref. N Engl J Med
285:267, July 29, 1971

360. NEW EVIDENCE INDICATES THAT PERINATAL TRANSMISSION IS AN IMPORTANT EPIDEMIOLOGIC FACTOR IN THE SPREAD OF CYTOMEGALOVIRUSES. POSTNATAL TRANSMISSION HAS BEEN DOCUMENTED FOR ALL OF THE FOLLOWING ROUTES, EXCEPT:

A. Fecal-oral
B. Organ transplantation
C. Breast milk
D. Blood transfusion
E. Saliva

Ref. N Engl J Med
285:268, July 29, 1971

FOOD POISONING

361. BACTERIAL CONTAMINATION OF AMERICA'S FOOD MAY RANK SECOND ONLY TO THE COMMON COLD AS A CAUSE OF ILLNESS. THE MOST COMMON CAUSE OF FOOD POISONING IN THIS COUNTRY IS:

A. Clostridium botulinum
B. Salmonella
C. Staphylococci
D. Vibrio parahemolyticus
E. Clostridium perfringens

Ref. Med World News
12:53, November 12, 1971

GRAFT VS. HOST DISEASE

362. PRELIMINARY OBSERVATIONS SUGGEST THAT WHEN BLOOD FROM A NON-HISTOCOMPATIBLE DONOR IS ADMINISTERED TO A CHILD WITH SWISS-TYPE AGAMMAGLOBULINEMIA GRAFT-VERSUS-HOST DISEASE MAY BE PREVENTED BY:

A. Using the mother as a donor
B. Corticosteroids
C. Massive doses of antibiotics
D. Irradiation of blood before transfusion
E. Using unmatched mitomycin-treated lymphocytes

Ref. JAMA
217:1037, August 23, 1971

DIAGNOSTIC PROBLEM

363. A 13 MONTH-OLD INFANT WITH AN UPPER RESPIRATORY TRACT INFECTION AND A TEMPERATURE OF 103° F., HAS A WARM TENDER PURPLISH-RED ERYSIPELOID LESION OF THE RIGHT CHEEK THAT LACKS A SHARPLY DEFINED BORDER. THE MOST LIKELY DIAGNOSIS IS:
A. Erythema infectiosum
B. Streptococcal cellulitis
C. Hemophilus influenzae, type b, cellulitis
D. Staphylococcal cellulitis
E. Pseudomonas cellulitis

Ref. Pediatr Clin N Am
17:415, May, 1970

HEPATITIS, SERUM, IMMUNIZATION

364. STUDIES OF ACTIVE IMMUNIZATION AGAINST VIRAL HEPATITIS, MS-2, TYPE B OR SERUM HEPATITIS HAVE DEMONSTRATED THE EFFECTIVENESS OF WHICH OF THE FOLLOWING IN PREVENTING THIS DISEASE:
A. Inoculation of boiled, inactivated MS-2 serum
B. Administration of standard human immune serum globulin
C. Parenteral attenuated MS-2 virus
D. Oral administration of MS-2 virus
E. Intranasal administration of MS-2 virus

Ref. JAMA
217:41, July 5, 1971

HERPES SIMPLEX, NEONATAL

365. IN HERPES SIMPLEX INFECTIONS OF THE NEWBORN INFANT ALL OF THE FOLLOWING ARE TRUE, EXCEPT:
A. Both strains of herpes simplex virus are capable of causing maternal vulvovaginitis
B. All neonatal herpetic infections which have been fatal have been associated with the type 2 strain
C. Transplacental infections with herpes simplex virus have been documented
D. The efficacy of cesarean section as a method of preventing neonatal infections is unproved
E. Present evidence suggests that transplacental type 1 herpes simplex antibodies do not afford protection, or lessen the illness of the newborn

Ref. J Pediatr
79:393, September, 1971

HERPES SIMPLEX, NEONATAL

366. HERPES SIMPLEX INFECTIONS OF THE NEWBORN INFANT ARE AN IMPORTANT CAUSE OF NEONATAL MORBIDITY AND MORTALITY. ALL OF THE FOLLOWING CLINICAL AND LABORATORY OBSERVATIONS HAVE BEEN CONFIRMED, EXCEPT:
A. There is an increased severity of herpes infections in premature infants
B. The spectrum of illness in the newborn may range from death to a complete and normal recovery
C. Disseminated intravascular coagulation has complicated neonatal herpes infections
D. The interferon system has been shown to be functional in the full-term newborn infant
E. Congenital herpes infections in the newborn have not occurred in the absence of a history of local lesions in the mother

Ref. J Pediatr
79:393, September, 1971

HERPESVIRUS

367. THE MOST COMMON EXAMPLE OF ENDOGENOUS RECURRENT VIRAL INFECTION IS REINFECTION DUE TO HERPES SIMPLEX VIRUS. EACH OF THE FOLLOWING STATEMENTS IN RECURRENT HERPES SIMPLEX INFECTIONS IS CORRECT, EXCEPT:

A. Most adult patients with herpes encephalitis have antibodies to herpesvirus suggesting endogenous reactivation of the virus
B. The presence of IgA and IgG in oral secretions to herpesvirus does not reduce the frequency of recurrence
C. The association of recurrent herpetic lesions and the fevers of malaria, pneumococcal and meningococcal infections is well known
D. Viral infections with fever are commonly associated with recurrent herpesvirus infections
E. Mensturation, corticosteroid administration and emotional stress may reactivate herpesvirus

Ref. N Engl J Med 284:766, April 8, 1971

HERPESVIRUS ENCEPHALITIS

368. HERPES HOMINIS ENCEPHALITIS IS THE MOST FREQUENT AND MOST DEVASTATING OF ACUTE VIRAL INFECTIONS OF THE BRAIN IN THE UNITED STATES TODAY. ALL OF THE FOLLOWING ARE CORRECT IN REGARD TO HERPES ENCEPHALITIS, EXCEPT:

A. Cutaneous herpetic lesions are present in most patients
B. Cerebrospinal fluid may be normal or may show only moderate numbers of lymphocytes
C. Benign aseptic meningitis may be caused by H. hominis
D. Some patients with encephalitis due to herpes simplex have prolonged courses that are difficult to distinguish from those of other children with subacute sclerosing panencephalitis
E. Antiherpesvirus antibodies may not be present in the spinal fluid of patients ill with herpes encephalitis

Ref. N Engl J Med 282:10, January 1, 1970

IMPETIGO, STREPTOCOCCAL

369. A VARIETY OF THERAPEUTIC REGIMENS ARE USED IN TREATING IMPETIGO, RANGING FROM THE REMOVAL OF CRUSTS AND CLEANSING WITH SOAP TO THE SYSTEMIC ADMINISTRATION OF ANTIBIOTICS. IN THE ASSESSMENT OF VARIOUS TREATMENT PROGRAMS IN EXPERIMENTAL INFECTION OF THE SKIN IN THE HAMSTER SIMULATING HUMAN IMPETIGO ALL OF THE FOLLOWING HAVE BEEN DEMONSTRATED, EXCEPT:

A. Scrubbing experimental impetigo with pHisoHex significantly delays healing and leads to the development of satellite lesions
B. The topical use of bacitracin ointment failed to demonstrate any benefits over untreated controls
C. The presence of penicillin-resistant staphylococci in human impetigo interferes with the effectiveness of penicillin therapy in staphylococcal-streptococcal mixed infections
D. Streptococci persist commonly in skin lesions for several days after the institution of systemic penicillin therapy
E. Whether penicillin treatment of impetigo due to nephritigenic strains will reduce the risk of acute nephritis is not known

Ref. Pediatrics 48:83, 1971

INFLUENZA VACCINE

370. RECENT STUDIES COMPARING THE ADMINISTRATION OF INFLUENZA VACCINE BY SUBCUTANEOUS, NASAL AND COMBINED ROUTES HAVE SUGGESTED ALL OF THE FOLLOWING, EXCEPT:

A. Parenteral vaccination provides sufficient secretory antibody to resist natural virus challenge on at least a temporary basis
B. Currently available influenza vaccines appear to protect civilian adults when given by the parenteral route
C. A standard dose of vaccine sprayed into the respiratory tract was not protective against the natural infection
D. Patients receiving vaccine by a combination of injection and nasal spray demonstrated significantly greater protection than those receiving parenteral vaccine alone
E. Natural influenza infection does not always stimulate "protective" antibody levels

Ref. Amer J Epidem 93:480, 1971

KVEIM TEST

371. THE CONCEPT THAT THE KVEIM TEST REPRESENTS A SPECIFIC HYPERSENSITIVITY RESPONSE TO SOME SUBSTANCE IN HUMAN SARCOIDAL TISSUE HAS BEEN CHALLENGED. EACH OF THE FOLLOWING OBSERVATIONS HAS BEEN MADE, EXCEPT:

A. The Kveim test appears to be an immunologic reaction associated with persistent lymphadenopathy of diverse causes
B. Typical reactions have been obtained in patients with chronic lymphatic leukemia, tuberculous adenitis and infectious mononucleosis
C. Kveim test responsiveness disappears when lymphadenopathy is gone
D. If lymph nodes are not enlarged in sarcoid the Kveim test tends to be negative irrespective of skin, liver, lung or bone involvement
E. The histology of the Kveim reaction closely resembles that of the tuberculin reaction and rarely have false positive or false negative reactions been a clinical problem

Ref. N Engl J Med 284:345, February 18, 1971

LISTERIA MONOCYTOGENES

372. BECAUSE OF ITS DIPHTHEROID-LIKE SHAPE, VARIATIONS IN MORPHOLOGY AND STAINING, AND BECAUSE OF ITS PRODUCTION OF BETA HEMOLYSIS, LISTERIA MONOCYTOGENES MAY BE OVERLOOKED IN CULTURES OF SPINAL FLUID. MENINGITIS CAUSED BY LISTERIA IS BEST TREATED WITH WHICH OF THE FOLLOWING ANTIBIOTICS IN TERMS OF EFFICACY AND TOXICITY?:

A. Ampicillin
B. Chloramphenicol
C. Tetracycline
D. Cephalothin
E. Kanamycin

Ref. N Engl J Med 285:598, September 9, 1971

MENINGOCOCCAL CARRIERS

373. WHEN EITHER RIFAMPIN, MINOCYCLINE OR AMPICILLIN ARE USED IN A MILITARY POPULATION TO TREAT THE MENINGOCOCCAL CARRIER ALL OF THE FOLLOWING ARE OBSERVED, EXCEPT:
A. The carrier rate returns rapidly to pretreatment levels with ampicillin
B. The majority of carriers treated with rifampin remain culture negative for as long as 30 days
C. The usefulness of rifampin in chemoprophylaxis is limited by the emergence of resistant strains
D. Rifampin is a more effective drug in the treatment of the carrier than minocycline because of greater concentrations in saliva
E. Rifampin does not always prevent the development of the carrier state when given to culture-negative military recruits

Ref. J Infect Dis
124:199, August, 1971

PARAINFLUENZA VIRUSES

374. PARAINFLUENZA VIRUSES ARE ASSOCIATED WITH ABOUT 8 PER CENT OF ALL ACUTE RESPIRATORY INFECTIONS IN CHILDREN ADMITTED TO THE HOSPITAL. ALL OF THE FOLLOWING ARE TRUE IN REGARD TO THESE IMPORTANT PATHOGENS, EXCEPT:
A. The clinical features of acute lower respiratory tract infection caused by parainfluenza virus type 3 are similar to those associated with the respiratory syncytial virus
B. Parainfluenza type 3 virus causes severe lower respiratory infections in infants under six months in contrast to type 1 and 2 infections
C. All three parainfluenza viruses may cause croup in those over 1 year of age
D. The respiratory syncytial virus is not associated with the croup syndrome in children
E. An effective method for the rapid diagnosis of parainfluenza virus infections by immunofluorescence has been devised using cells from nasopharyngeal secretions

Ref. Br Med J
2:7, April 3, 1971

PARAPERTUSSIS

375. TWENTY YEARS'OBSERVATIONS IN DENMARK OF EPIDEMICS OF PARAPERTUSSIS HAVE SHOWN ALL OF THE FOLLOWING, EXCEPT:
A. Parapertussis is as widespread as pertussis in densely populated areas
B. Infections with parapertussis without symptoms are most uncommon
C. The amount of heat-labile toxin produced by Bord. pertussis is greater than that produced by Bord. parapertussis, which may account for the greater intensity of clinical manifestations
D. Both infections present with epidemics every fourth year with a two year shift between the pertussis and parapertussis peaks
E. Pertussis vaccination may influence the clinical course of parapertussis, although it does not prevent infection

Ref. Lancet
1:1195, June 12, 1971

PSEUDOMONAS SEPSIS

376. EMPIRIC THERAPY WITH CARBENICILLIN AND GENTAMICIN FOR FEBRILE PATIENTS WITH CANCER AND GRANULOCYTOPENIA HAS LED TO AN INCREASED SURVIVAL IN INFECTIONS WITH PSEUDOMONAS AERUGINOSA. EACH OF THE FOLLOWING HAS BEEN SUGGESTED IN THIS DIFFICULT PROBLEM IN PATIENTS WITH IMPAIRED HOST RESISTANCE, EXCEPT:

A. Carbenicillin and gentamicin should be administered intermittently and never mixed for intravenous use
B. Carbenicillin resembles ampicillin in its spectrum but has additional effectiveness for indole-positive proteus strains as well as for most isolates of pseudomonas aeruginosa
C. Superinfection is a rare clinical event when combined antibiotic therapy is given
D. Carbenicillin is often ineffective against members of the klebsiella-enterobacter-serratia group
E. Gentamicin is broadly effective against aerobic gram-negative organisms

Ref. N Engl J Med 284:1061, May 13, 1971

RABIES

377. THE PREVENTION OF RABIES BY IMMUNOLOGIC MEANS IS PRESENTLY IN AN UNSATISFACTORY STATE. EACH OF THE FOLLOWING IS CORRECT, EXCEPT:

A. The risk of allergic encephalomyelitis is greater with the Semple inactivated rabies vaccine than with the Duck embryo vaccine
B. Antibody titers are lower following the use of the Duck embryo vaccine than with the Semple vaccine
C. Human rabies-immune globulin has not been shown to be effective in protection tests
D. Thorough cleaning of a wound infected with rabies virus with virucidal solutions is equal in importance to the use of vaccine and antiserum
E. The treatment of neurologic reactions to rabies vaccine includes the use of steroids

Ref. J Infect Dis 123:235, February, 1971

378. THE BITE OF AN ANIMAL IS NOT AUTOMATICALLY REASON FOR VACCINATION AGAINST RABIES. OVER ONE-HALF MILLION DOSES OF RABIES VACCINES ARE ADMINISTERED ANNUALLY IN THE UNITED STATES. EACH OF THE FOLLOWING IS CORRECT IN REGARD TO RABIES, EXCEPT:

A. Whiskeys of 86 proof or greater can be used in emergencies to treat animal bites in humans
B. Rodent bites, such as those inflicted on slum children by rats often present a potential for rabies infection
C. Strains of rabies virus developed for vaccination of dogs, when given to other species, may not be sufficiently attenuated. Rabies may be provoked in a pet rodent, resulting in a hazard for human contacts
D. Bites of sylvatic animals, when unprovoked, must be considered contaminated by rabies virus unless the biting animal can be captured and shown to be free of rabies
E. Antiserum should be used locally and parenterally in addition to vaccine whenever exposure to rabies has been proven or is highly likely

Ref. J Infect Dis 123:227, February, 1971

RECURRENT VIRAL INFECTIONS

379. RECURRENT VIRAL INFECTION OR REINFECTION REPRESENTS AN INFECTION IN CHILDREN WITH PARTIAL IMMUNITY FROM PREVIOUS EXPERIENCE WITH THE SAME VIRUS. EACH OF THE FOLLOWING STATEMENTS IS CORRECT, EXCEPT:

A. Reinfection with varicella-zoster virus is characterized by neurotransmission after reactivation of the virus which has probably been in a latent state in a dorsal root ganglion
B. Reinfection with cytomegalovirus occurs in those receiving immunosuppressive therapy
C. Exogenous reinfection by respiratory viruses is common
D. Reinfection by serum hepatitis virus has been demonstrated in drug addicts
E. Reinfection by specific viruses results usually in a more severe clinical expression

Ref. N Engl J Med 284:768, April 8, 1971

RESPIRATORY SYNCYTIAL VIRUS VACCINE

380. A FOLLOW-UP OF THE CHILDREN WHO HAD BEEN IMMUNIZED WITH A KILLED RESPIRATORY SYNCYTIAL VIRUS VACCINE HAS RESULTED IN AN ATYPICAL DISEASE WHEN PATIENTS HAVE BEEN INFECTED WITH THE NATURAL VIRUS. EACH OF THE FOLLOWING IS CORRECT, EXCEPT:

A. A predisposition prevails in vaccinees to a more severe lower respiratory tract disease from the respiratory syncytial virus for at least four years after vaccination
B. A rash often accompanies the atypical disease seen in vaccinees
C. Eosinophilia has been commonly observed in the atypical disease
D. Bronchopneumonia has been seen in all children, sometimes with a pleural effusion
E. The atypical disease, as with its natural counterpart, has been unresponsive to steroids

Ref. Infect Dis Sect Proceedings of APS/SPR, April 30, 1971

ROCKY MOUNTAIN SPOTTED FEVER

381. IN 1969 THERE WAS MORE THAN A 50 PER CENT INCREASE IN THE REPORTED INCIDENCE OF TICK-BORNE TYPHUS (ROCKY MOUNTAIN SPOTTED FEVER) IN THE U.S.A. ALL OF THE FOLLOWING ARE TRUE IN REGARD TO THIS POTENTIALLY FATAL DISEASE, EXCEPT:

A. For many years this has been primarily a disease of the south-atlantic and south-central states and is now relatively rare in the mountain states
B. The American dog tick, Dermacentor variabilis, is the only recognized vector of the disease
C. Conclusive laboratory diagnosis cannot generally be made until convalescence
D. The complement-fixation test is more specific than the Proteus agglutinins
E. An infected tick must be warmed or must ingest a fresh blood meal to "reactivate the rickettsia"

Ref. JAMA 216:1003, May 10, 1971

RUBELLA

382. REINFECTION BY THE RUBELLA VIRUS HAS BEEN STUDIED INTENSIVELY BECAUSE OF THE WIDESPREAD USE OF THE RUBELLA VACCINE. EACH OF THE FOLLOWING STATEMENTS IS CORRECT, EXCEPT:

A. After the use of the Cendehill vaccine the frequency of reinfection after vaccination in closed communities has varied from 50 to 84 per cent
B. Reinfection after the natural disease is much less frequent
C. Viremia has not been detected in immune subjects
D. Viral excretion can be demonstrated in vaccine-immune children after challange with the wild rubella virus
E. There is strong evidence to suggest that an immune pregnant woman can transmit congenital rubella after a clinically inapparent reinfection

Ref. N Engl J Med
284:769, April 8, 1971

RUBELLA IMMUNE GLOBULIN

383. DESPITE THE WIDE USE OF RUBELLA VIRUS VACCINE THE NEED FOR AN EFFECTIVE PASSIVE MEANS OF IMMUNIZATION STILL EXISTS. STUDIES OF A HIGH TITER ANTIRUBELLA HUMAN IMMUNOGLOBULIN HAVE SHOWN ALL OF THE FOLLOWING (AFTER THE CHALLENGE OF INTRANASAL LIVE RUBELLA VIRUS), EXCEPT:

A. A depression of pharyngeal shedding of live virus
B. Decreased incidence of viremia
C. Prevention of seroconversion
D. A prolongation of the incubation period
E. An inability to prevent the rash in all

Ref. Infect Dis Sect,
Proceedings of APS/SPR,
April 30, 1971

RUBELLA VACCINE AND THE ARM SYNDROME

384. FOLLOWING COMMUNITY RUBELLA IMMUNIZATION PROGRAMS FOR CHILDREN CURIOUS NEW "PAIN SYNDROMES" HAVE BEEN DESCRIBED. EACH OF THE FOLLOWING IS CORRECT IN REGARD TO THE "ARM SYNDROME," EXCEPT:

A. The children characteristically awaken at night with pain in both wrists and hands
B. Paresthesias in the hands and fingers are common
C. No joint swelling, tenderness or limitation of motion is usually found
D. Younger children have been noted by their parents frequently to rub their hands as though they itch
E. Nerve conduction tests are normal

Ref. JAMA
214:2287, December 28, 1970

RUBELLA VACCINE AND THE LEG SYNDROME

385. THE "LEG SYNDROME" HAS BEEN DESCRIBED FOLLOWING RUBELLA VIRUS VACCINATION IN CHILDREN. EACH OF THE FOLLOWING STATEMENTS IS CORRECT, EXCEPT:

A. The syndrome is characterized by recurrences
B. All children have complained of pain localized to the popliteal fossa
C. In contrast to the "Arm syndrome" pain is most pronounced on awakening in the morning and diminished during the day
D. The typical stance of an affected child resembles a "baseball catcher's crouch"
E. Signs of joint inflammation are consistently present

Ref. JAMA
214:2290, December 28, 1970

RUBELLA VIRUS VACCINE

386. LIVE, ATTENUATED RUBELLA VIRUS VACCINE APPEARS TO BE A HIGHLY EFFECTIVE IMMUNIZING AGENT AND THE FIRST SUITABLE METHOD OF CONTROLLING RUBELLA. EACH OF THE FOLLOWING IS CORRECT, EXCEPT:

A. Rubella-like symptoms of rash and lymphadenopathy occur occasionally after vaccination
B. Arthralgia and arthritis has occurred more frequently following the use of the more immunogenic canine renal cell vaccine
C. Vaccinees may shed relatively small amounts of virus from the pharynx for brief periods between the first and fourth weeks after inoculation
D. The use of rubella vaccine in children whose mothers are pregnant is contraindicated
E. Vaccinees exposed to rubella often develop increases in antibody titers without clinical symptoms

Ref. Recommendation of the Public Health Service Advisory Committee on Immunization Practices
Rubella Virus Vaccine
August 29, 1970

RUBELLA VACCINE AND ARTHRITIS

387. ARTHRITIS AFTER RUBELLA VACCINATION IS DISTRESSING AND MAY LEAD TO UNNECESSARY LABORATORY INVESTIGATION. EACH OF THE FOLLOWING IS CORRECT, EXCEPT:

A. Arthritis may occur nearly two months after vaccination
B. The sedimentation rate in rubella vaccine associated arthritis is usually normal
C. Rubella vaccine virus has been recovered from synovial fluid
D. Serum sickness is suggested by the other manifestations seen in rubella vaccine virus arthritis
E. Definite evidence of joint effusion is not usually seen

Ref. Arthritis Rheum
14:19, January, February, 1971

RUBELLA VACCINE AND PREGNANCY

388. THE NEED FOR EXTREME CAUTION IN VACCINATING POSTPUBERTAL WOMEN WITH ATTENUATED RUBELLA VIRUS STILL EXISTS. DESPITE CURRENT RECOMMENDATIONS HUNDREDS OF WOMEN AND ADOLESCENT GIRLS HAVE BEEN INOCULATED WHEN PREGNANT. EACH OF THE FOLLOWING IS CORRECT, EXCEPT:
A. There is at present no definitive information concerning the teratogenic potential of attenuated rubella virus vaccines
B. Attenuated virus can produce a chronic placental infection
C. Virus has not been recovered from the fetus after the administration of the rubella vaccine to the mother
D. The relative risks of vaccination as compared to natural rubella during pregnancy are unknown
E. The viremia of natural rubella infection sometimes fails to spread from the mother to the conceptus

Ref. N Engl J Med 284:870, April 22, 1971

COMBINED RUBEOLA-RUBELLA-MUMPS VACCINE

389. THE COMBINED USE OF THE LIVE MEASLES (MORATEN), RUBELLA (HPV-77 DUCK), AND MUMPS (JERYL LYNN) VIRUSES IN ONE VACCINE HAS SHOWN ALL OF THE FOLLOWING, EXCEPT:
A. Sero-conversion rates in excess of 90 per cent
B. An increased incidence of febrile responses in contrast to the individual vaccines
C. A remarkable freedom from interference
D. Mean antibody titers which are the same as when used individually
E. A method of conserving medical manhours which should receive general acceptance

Ref. JAMA 218:57, October 4, 1971

SMALLPOX VACCINATION, COMPLICATIONS

390. ABOUT HALF OF 68 DEATHS FROM COMPLICATIONS OF SMALLPOX VACCINATION OVER A 9 YEAR PERIOD IN THE USA RESULTED FROM:
A. Postvaccinal encephalomyelitis
B. Eczema vaccinatum
C. Progressive vaccinia
D. Generalized vaccinia
E. Hypersensitivity reactions (Stevens-Johnson syndrome)

Ref. JAMA 212:441, 1970

SPOROTRICHOSIS

391. SPOROTRICHOSIS SHOULD BE SUGGESTED BY ALL OF THE FOLLOWING CLINICAL CHARACTERISTICS, EXCEPT:
A. Oral potassium iodide therapy is curative
B. Scarring does not occur at the site of the primary lesion
C. Visible lymphangitic spread from the primary ulcer is common
D. The primary ulcer is most apt to occur on exposed surfaces and is non-tender
E. Sporothrix schenckii is found on many forms of vegetation and does not seem capable of penetrating intact skin

Ref. Am J Dis Child 122:325, October, 1971

STREPTOCOCCAL PHARYNGITIS

392. CROWDED LIVING CONDITIONS PROMOTE THE EPIDEMIC SPREAD OF STREPTOCOCCAL PHARYNGITIS AND ENHANCE THE RISK OF RHEUMATIC FEVER IN CHILDHOOD. EACH OF THE FOLLOWING STATEMENTS IN REGARD TO STREPTOCOCCAL DISEASE IS CORRECT, EXCEPT:

A. Penicillinase-producing staphylococci account for a significant number of treatment failures
B. Dramatic symptomatic relief of streptococcal sore throat follows the institution of penicillin therapy
C. Isolation of streptococci on throat culture does not establish causation
D. Treatment failure is often linked to compliance, particularly, in low income populations
E. Bacterial recurrence rates after appropriate penicillin therapy are discouragingly high, ranging from 7 to 25 per cent

Ref. Pediatr Clin N Am
18:145, February, 1971

STREPTOCOCCAL PHARYNGITIS

393. THE ACCURATE DIAGNOSIS OF STREPTOCOCCAL PHARYNGITIS IS OF IMPORTANCE IN ANY PROGRAM DESIGNED TO PREVENT RHEUMATIC FEVER. THE DEMONSTRATION OF THE ORGANISM BY THROAT CULTURE IS ESSENTIAL FOR AN ACCURATE DIAGNOSIS. EACH OF THE FOLLOWING STATEMENTS REGARDING STREPTOCOCCAL PHARYNGITIS IS CORRECT, EXCEPT:

A. Mild cases of streptococcal pharyngitis may be followed by rheumatic fever
B. The identification of organisms other than streptococci is unnecessary since only gonococci, corynebacterium diphtheriae and perhaps the organisms of Vincent's angina are capable of causing pharyngitis
C. Streptococci survive for days and even weeks on dried swabs
D. It is unnecessary to use sheep blood agar and outdated human blood should be utilized in preparing culture media as an economy measure to identify streptococci
E. Presumptive identification of Group A streptococci may be provided by the selective inhibition of such strains by bacitracin

Ref. Pediatr Clin N Am
18:125, February, 1971

STREPTOCOCCAL DISEASE

394. ASSUMING THAT DOSAGE IS PROPER FOR AGE AND WEIGHT WHICH OF THE FOLLOWING REGIMENS REPRESENTS INADEQUATE THERAPY FOR GROUP A BETA HEMOLYTIC STREPTOCOCCAL PHARYNGITIS IN A 5 YEAR-OLD GIRL?:

A. Oral ampicillin for 10 days
B. Oral penicillin G for 10 days
C. Oral erythromycin for 10 days
D. One intramuscular injection of benzathine penicillin
E. One intramuscular injection of procaine penicillin

Ref. J Pediatr
75:923, December, 1969

STREPTOCOCCAL ANTIBODIES

395. DETERMINATIONS OF STREPTOCOCCAL ANTIBODIES ARE USEFUL TESTS TO DOCUMENT A RECENT STREPTOCOCCAL INFECTION. EACH OF THE FOLLOWING STATEMENTS IS CORRECT, EXCEPT:
A. Results obtained from the ASO and the newer anti-DNA-se B tests are remarkably reproducible when properly performed
B. ASO titers of 250 or greater are commonly found in "normal" children living in slum areas of the great cities
C. An elevated titer of streptococcal antibodies is best found about two weeks after the infection
D. A high ASO titer is a decisive argument in favor of a diagnosis of rheumatic fever
E. Low titers of streptococcal antibodies are usually found in Sydenham's chorea probably owing to a longer latent period of this manifestation

Ref. Pediatr Clin N Am 18:136, February, 1971

SYPHILIS AND SEROLOGY

396. THE MOST SENSITIVE TEST AVAILABLE IN ALL STAGES OF SYPHILIS, BUT ONE WHICH MAY HAVE FALSE-POSITIVE REACTIONS IN CHILDREN WITH INCREASED OR ABNORMAL GLOBULINS IS:
A. FTA-ABS (Fluorescent treponemal antibody absorption)
B. VDRL
C. Kolmer complement-fixation
D. Hinton
E. TPI (T. pallidum immobilization)

Ref. N Engl J Med 284:642, March 25, 1971

TOXOPLASMA GONDII

397. FROM THE FECES OF WHICH OF THE FOLLOWING HOUSEHOLD PETS HAS THE RESISTANT OOCYST STAGE OF TOXOPLASMA GONDII BEEN ISOLATED SUGGESTING A BASIC MEANS BY WHICH THE PARASITE IS MAINTAINED AND DISSEMINATED?:
A. Parakeet
B. Turtle
C. Dog
D. Cat
E. Tropical fish

Ref. J Infect Dis 124:227, August, 1971

TUBERCULOSIS

398. THE INTERPRETATION OF CHEST ROENTGENOGRAMS IS AN IMPORTANT CONSIDERATION IN THE DIAGNOSIS OF TUBERCULOUS MENINGITIS. THE MOST COMMON FINDING IN A CHEST X-RAY IN CHILDREN ILL WITH TUBERCULOUS MENINGITIS IS:
A. Normal chest
B. Primary complex
C. Disseminated miliary tuberculosis
D. Miliary pattern with primary complex
E. Calcifying primary intrathoracic tuberculosis

Ref. Amer J Dis Child 121:389, May, 1971

TUBERCULOSIS, BCG

399. CHILDREN BORN OF TUBERCULOUS MOTHERS HAVE THE HIGHEST RISK OF BECOMING INFECTED, AND THE POOREST PROGNOSIS SHOULD THEY ACQUIRE THE DISEASE. WHICH OF THE FOLLOWING PROGRAMS HAS HAD THE MOST SUCCESS IN THE PREVENTION OF TUBERCULOSIS IN INFANTS AT RISK AT BIRTH?:

A. BCG vaccination
B. Observation of the infant with periodic chest X-rays and tuberculin testing
C. Gross and histologic examination of the placenta before the use of isoniazid in the infant
D. Isolation of the infant until the mother is no longer considered to be infectious
E. Isoniazid prophylaxis for a one-year period

Ref. Clin Pediatr
9:632, November, 1970

TUBERCULIN TESTING

400. WHEN PROPERLY USED, THE TUBERCULIN TEST REPRESENTS THE MOST RELIABLE METHOD FOR THE DETECTION OF CHILDHOOD TUBERCULOSIS. ALL OF THE FOLLOWING STATEMENTS ARE CORRECT, EXCEPT:

A. Tuberculin hypersensitivity may be temporarily suppressed (weeks) after immunization with live measles vaccine
B. The extent of a tuberculin reaction is an accurate index of the presence or absence of activity of a tuberculous lesion
C. The second-strength PPD has little or no value when screening for tuberculosis in essentially healthy children
D. When a child exhibits a negative reaction to intermediate strength PPD and a positive reaction to second-strength PPD, one must exclude atypical mycobacterial disease
E. A negative intermediate-strength PPD cannot be relied upon to exclude tuberculosis in clinically ill patients

Ref. N Engl J Med
285:294, July 29, 1971

401. TYPHOID CARRIERS

ALTHOUGH THE INCIDENCE OF TYPHOID FEVER HAS DECLINED IN THE U.S.A. ABOUT 700 ISOLATIONS ARE REPORTED EACH YEAR TO THE CENTER FOR DISEASE CONTROL. EACH OF THE FOLLOWING STATEMENTS IS CORRECT, EXCEPT:

A. Adults become chronic carriers much more frequently than do children after the acute infection
B. Chloramphenicol is the drug of choice in acute typhoid fever
C. Ampicillin appears to be the drug by choice for the treatment of chronic typhoid carriers
D. The presence or absence of gallbladder disease does not influence the outcome of therapy with ampicillin in the carrier
E. Salmonella typhosa is unlike other salmonellas in that the reservoir is the human patient or carrier

Ref. J Infect Dis
125:170, February, 1972

VARICELLA

402. VARICELLA IS A BENIGN ILLNESS FOR MOST CHILDREN. FOR SOME, HOWEVER, IT MAY BE A SEVERE OR FATAL EXPERIENCE. EACH OF THE FOLLOWING STATEMENTS IS CORRECT REGARDING SUSCEPTIBLE CHILDREN WHO ARE EXPOSED TO CHICKENPOX, EXCEPT:

A. The administration of herpes zoster immune globulin will prevent chickenpox
B. Passive immunization with human immune serum globulin does not protect children from chickenpox
C. Massive doses of human immune serum globulin (0.6 ml per pound of body weight) regularly prevent chickenpox
D. Newborn infants are at serious risk in some instances from chickenpox
E. The use of herpes zoster immune globulin is indicated in children who are receiving antimetabolites

Ref. J Infect Dis
125:82, January, 1972

VENEZUELAN EQUINE ENCEPHALOMYELITIS

403. IN THE SPRING AND SUMMER OF 1971 CONSIDERABLE ANXIETY WAS GENERATED OVER AN OUTBREAK OF VENEZUELAN EQUINE ENCEPHALOMYELITIS (VEE) WHICH KILLED HUNDREDS OF HORSES IN THE SOUTHWEST. YOU WOULD HAVE SUGGESTED ALL OF THE FOLLOWING TO YOUR PATIENTS, EXCEPT:

A. Widespread clinical use of the live virus vaccine is not recommended for humans
B. VEE is a deadly disease in horses
C. The vaccine has demonstrated side-effects in humans, such as fever and headache
D. Although the number of cases of VEE in humans has been relatively small and the mortality low, serious neurologic sequellae were common
E. The primary disease vector appears to be the mosquito

Ref. JAMA
217:758, August 9, 1971

FOR EACH OF THE FOLLOWING QUESTIONS, SELECT THE ONE MOST APPROPRIATE ANSWER BY USING THE KEY OUTLINED BELOW:

1. If A, B and C are correct
2. If A and C are correct
3. If B and D are correct
4. If all are correct
5. If all are incorrect

MYCOPLASMAS

404. ALTHOUGH THEY HAVE BEEN CALLED "JOKERS IN THE MICROBIOLOGIC PACK" ADDITIONAL EVIDENCE SUGGESTS A RELATIONSHIP OF T-STRAIN MYCOPLASMAS TO WHICH OF THE FOLLOWING?:

A. Non-gonococcal urethritis
B. Sexual exposure
C. Low birth weight infants
D. Gastroenteritis
E. Urinary tract infection

Ref. N Engl J Med
284:167, January 28, 1971
Med World News
13:38, February 4, 1972

AMPICILLIN AND MENINGITIS

405. FACTORS WHICH MAY CONTRIBUTE TO THE PERSISTENCE OR RELAPSE OF INFECTION IN HEMOPHILUS INFLUENZA, TYPE B MENINGITIS TREATED WITH AMPICILLIN SODIUM HAVE INCLUDED:
A. Infection of the subdural space
B. Use of the intramuscular route of administration
C. Presence of ventriculitis and hydrocephalus
D. Development of resistance to ampicillin by the organism
E. Demonstration that ampicillin penetration in brain tissue in meningitis is poor

Ref. Am J Dis Child 122:328, October, 1971

ANTIBIOTICS AND PARENTERAL SOLUTIONS

406. WHICH OF THE FOLLOWING ANTIBIOTICS WHEN ADDED TO A VARIETY OF PARENTERAL SOLUTIONS PROVED TO BE STABLE AT ALL TEMPERATURES DURING A 24-HOUR OBSERVATION PERIOD?:
A. Carbenicillin
B. Methicillin
C. Penicillin G
D. Cephalothin
E. Kanamycin

Ref. Pediatrics 49:22, January, 1972

ASPERGILLUS

407. ASPERGILLUS FUMIGATUS HAS BEEN ASSOCIATED WITH WHICH OF THE FOLLOWING IN MAN?:
A. Respiratory tract contaminant
B. Saprophyte in tuberculous or histoplasmic cavities
C. Allergen with pulmonary infiltrates ("fungus balls")
D. Invasive pathogen in patients receiving immunosuppressive therapy
E. Hyphae in the muscular walls of arteries serving to sustain disseminated intravascular coagulation

Ref. Arch Intern Med 128:790, 1971

CANDIDIASIS, RENAL

408. RENAL INVOLVEMENT IN SYSTEMIC CANDIDIASIS IS COMMON AND IS ASSOCIATED WITH WHICH OF THE FOLLOWING?:
A. Roentgenographic evidence of smooth or shaggy lucent-filling defects in the renal calyces or pelvis
B. Acute renal failure
C. Obstruction of the renal pelvis and ureter by mycelial "balls"
D. Papillary necrosis
E. Cortical and medullary abscesses

Ref. Radiology 101:567, December, 1971

CANDIDA, SYSTEMIC

409. DEEP FUNGAL INFECTIONS IN THE COMPROMISED HOST ARE MOST FREQUENTLY RELATED TO CANDIDA SPECIES. THE DIAGNOSIS OF SYSTEMIC CANDIDIASIS IS MOST STRONGLY SUGGESTED BY WHICH OF THE FOLLOWING?:

A. Microscopic demonstration of pseudohyphae and blastospores in smears of peripheral blood
B. Precipitin test
C. Blood cultures
D. Direct examination of fresh urine
E. Stool cultures

Ref. N Engl J Med
285:1010, October 28, 1971
J Infect Dis
125:190, February, 1972

EPIGLOTTITIS

410. EPIGLOTTITIS IS A SERIOUS EMERGENCY OF THE AIRWAY IN CHILDREN AND ASSOCIATED WITH WHICH OF THE FOLLOWING?:

A. Respiratory distress for more than 12 hours
B. Usually seen under 2 years of age
C. Change in voice or hoarseness frequently present
D. Tracheostomy seldom indicated
E. Lateral neck X-rays necessary for diagnosis

Ref. Pediatr Clin N Am
17:415, May, 1970
Br Med J
1:40, 1972

EXANTHEMS AND VIRUS ISOLATION

411. IT IS THOUGHT THAT THE RASH ASSOCIATED WITH MANY VIRAL DISEASES RESULTS FROM DERMAL INJURY FROM THE REPLICATION OF VIRUS WITHIN SKIN CELLS, PERHAPS IN COMBINATION WITH AN IMMUNOLOGIC REACTION AGAINST VIRAL ANTIGEN DEPOSITED IN THE SKIN. FROM WHICH OF THE FOLLOWING EXANTHEMS HAS VIRUS BEEN RECOVERED FROM SKIN CULTURES?:

A. Vaccinia
B. Varicella
C. Herpes simplex
D. Congenital rubella
E. Rubella

Ref. N Engl J Med
285:664, September 16, 1971

HEPATITIS, SERUM GLOBULIN

412. CLINICAL INVESTIGATIONS WITH THE USE OF "SERUM HEPATITIS IMMUNE GLOBULIN" IN THE PREVENTION, MODIFICATION AND TREATMENT OF SERUM HEPATITIS HAVE SUGGESTED WHICH OF THE FOLLOWING?:

A. Passive immunity in the presence of infection with the A or infectious hepatitis virus usually results in long lasting immunity
B. Small amounts of gamma globulin prepared so that it may be used intravenously, when added to whole blood before transfusion, may neutralize or modify the hepatitis virus
C. An increased frequency of chronic carriers may result from the use of "serum hepatitis immune globulin"
D. The potential for producing chronic liver disease from the suppression of immune responses is a theoretical risk from the use of "serum hepatitis immune globulin"
E. Serum hepatitis antibody titers tend to be higher in paid blood donors

Ref. N Engl J Med
285:933, October 21, 1971

HEPATITIS, CHRONIC

413. ALTHOUGH THE DEFINITION OF ACTIVE CHRONIC HEPATITIS IS ONE OF MANY UNANSWERED QUESTIONS, WHICH OF THE FOLLOWING STATEMENTS ARE CORRECT IN REGARD TO THE USE OF CORTICOSTEROIDS IN THIS PROBLEM?:

A. Corticosteroid therapy inhibits immune and inflammatory mechanisms associated with chronic "lupoid" hepatitis
B. Steroid therapy is associated with improved mortality in the first 6 months in chronic "lupoid" hepatitis
C. Whether or not steroid therapy prevents progression to cirrhosis is not fully substantiated
D. No firm guidelines exist for the use of steroids in chronic hepatitis associated with the hepatitis-associated antigen (H. A. A.)
E. Although fetal loss is high, transplacental spread of liver disease does not occur in chronic "lupoid" hepatitis

Ref. Quarterly J Med
40:159, 1971

HEPATITIS, SERUM, TRANSMISSION

414. THE TRANSMISSION OF VIRAL HEPATITIS, TYPE B (AUSTRALIA ANTIGEN-ASSOCIATED SERUM HEPATITIS) APPEARS TO BE POSSIBLE BY WHICH OF THE FOLLOWING, EXCEPT?:

A. Blood transfusion
B. Fecal-oral
C. Skin abrasions
D. Bleeding gums and poor dental hygiene
E. Sexual contact

Ref. N Engl J Med
285:1363, December 9, 1971

INFLUENZA AND AMANTADINE

415. IMMUNIZATION AND THE USE OF AMANTADINE IN THE CONTROL OF INFLUENZA HAVE BEEN ASSOCIATED WITH WHICH OF THE FOLLOWING?:

A. Immunization with influenza virus vaccine gives an immune response which equals that of natural infection
B. Amantadine inhibits the escape of virus from infected cells
C. Amantadine has been proven effective in the treatment of influenza although its effect on fever has not been statistically significant
D. In the treatment of influenza the use of amantadine for periods of two to three weeks has been associated with significant toxicity
E. Amantadine is effective in vitro and in vivo against all strains of influenza virus

Ref. N Engl J Med
285:1260, November 25, 1971

MEASLES, ATYPICAL

416. SEVERE ATYPICAL MEASLES MAY RESULT FROM EXPOSURE TO NATURAL MEASLES SEVERAL YEARS AFTER RECEIVING TWO OR MORE INJECTIONS OF THE INACTIVATED VACCINE. THE RASH DIFFERS FROM UNMODIFIED MEASLES IN WHICH OF THE FOLLOWING CHARACTERISTICS?:

A. A mixture of papular, petechial, vesicular and urticarial lesions
B. Progression toward the head instead of away from it
C. Most dense in the lower limbs and in creases
D. Association with edema of the limbs
E. Onset around the feet instead of hairline

Ref. Br Med J
2:235, May, 1971
Acta Paediatrica Japonica
13:26, June, 1971

MENINGITIS, NEONATAL

417. NEONATAL MENINGITIS HAS AN ASSOCIATION WITH WHICH OF THE FOLLOWING COMPLICATIONS OF PREGNANCY AND DELIVERY?:

A. Fetal distress
B. Prenatal pneumonia
C. Prematurity
D. Maternal urinary tract infection
E. Premature rupture of membranes

Ref. Br Med J
4:318, November, 1970

MENINGITIS, BACTERIAL, PROLONGED FEVER

418. FEVER IN BACTERIAL MENINGITIS MAY PERSIST IN SOME CHILDREN WHO ARE OTHERWISE CLINICALLY RECOVERED FROM THEIR ILLNESS, OR IT MAY RECUR DURING TREATMENT AFTER DEFERVESCENCE WITHOUT EVIDENCE THAT THE MENINGITIS HAS BECOME ACTIVE AGAIN. WHICH OF THE FOLLOWING ARE MOST LIKELY TO BE ASSOCIATED WITH BRINGING ABOUT RAPID SUBSIDENCE OF FEVER IN SUCH PATIENTS?:

A. Subdural taps
B. Removing the intravenous catheter
C. Changing the antibiotic
D. Stopping the antibiotic
E. Adding intrathecal antibiotics

Ref. Br Med J
1:474, February, 27, 1971

NEONATAL MENINGITIS

419. THE EARLY CLINICAL PICTURE OF MENINGITIS IN THE NEWBORN IS CHARACTERIZED BY WHICH OF THE FOLLOWING CLINICAL SIGNS?:
A. Opisthotonus
B. Bulging fontanelle
C. Nuchal rigidity
D. Coma
E. Convulsions

Ref. Br Med J
4:319, November 7, 1970

MENINGITIS, H. INFLUENZA

420. IN A COMPARATIVE STUDY OF AMPICILLIN AND CHLORAMPHENICOL IN THE TREATMENT OF HEMOPHILUS INFLUENZAE MENINGITIS WHICH OF THE FOLLOWING WERE OBSERVED IN THE AMPICILLIN TREATED GROUP?:
A. Fewer subdural effusions
B. A more prolonged febrile course
C. Decreased mortality
D. A similar incidence of neurological sequelae
E. Slower clinical response (CSF culture and sugar)

Ref. Pediatrics
48:411, September, 1971

MYCOBACTERIA, ATYPICAL

421. ANONYMOUS MYCOBACTERIA ARE BEING ISOLATED WITH INCREASING FREQUENCY FROM LYMPH NODES IN CHILDREN. WHICH OF THE FOLLOWING STATEMENTS ARE APPLICABLE TO INFECTIONS WITH THESE ORGANISMS?:
A. Isolation of the child is unnecessary
B. Excision of infected nodes is the treatment of choice
C. Involvement of the tonsillar and submandibular lymph nodes are the most common sites of infection
D. Chemotherapy is not required and is of little value
E. Contamination of the wound during excision by liquefied or caseous materials seldom interferes with primary healing

Ref. Austr Pediatr J
7:97, June, 1971

PLAGUE AND THE HOUSEHOLD PET

422. ONE OF THE PROBLEMS IN THE IDENTIFICATION OF FOCI OF PLAGUE HAS RESTED WITH THE ISOLATION OF YERSINIA PESTIS FROM RODENTS OR THEIR FLEAS. WHICH OF THE FOLLOWING ARE NEWLY DISCOVERED EPIDEMIOLOGIC FACTS?:
A. Dogs in an endemic area of plague are often sero-positive
B. Plague appears to be a mild disease for the household dog
C. Cats are infected frequently under natural circumstances as a result of contact with plague-infected rodents or their fleas
D. Both dogs and cats are susceptible to experimental plague infection
E. Plague-infected fleas have been collected from both dogs and cats

Ref. J Infect Dis
124:522, November, 1971

PSEUDOMONAS INFECTIONS

423. PSEUDOMONAS AERUGINOSA INFECTIONS HAVE INCREASED IN FREQUENCY IN RECENT YEARS AND HAVE BEEN COMMONLY ASSOCIATED WITH WHICH OF THE FOLLOWING ENTITIES?:
A. Leukemia
B. Thymic aplasia
C. Extensive thermal burns
D. Inhalation therapy equipment
E. Cystic fibrosis

Ref. JAMA
218:62, October 4, 1971

SHIGELLA

424. SHIGELLA INFECTIONS:
A. Have been associated with "rose spots"
B. Usually are associated with family or institutional outbreaks
C. Are not uncommonly manifest at the onset by a generalized seizure
D. Are transmitted frequently by pets such as turtles
E. Are often traced to contaminated meat and poultry products

Ref. Am J Dis Child
119:152, February, 1970

STAPHYLOCOCCUS AUREUS 502A

425. ALTHOUGH THE RISK OF SERIOUS INFECTION DUE TO STAPHYLOCOCCUS AUREUS 502A IS LOW WHEN IT IS USED TO ABORT EPIDEMICS OF STAPHYLOCOCCAL DISEASE WHICH OF THE FOLLOWING HAVE BEEN DESCRIBED AS COMPLICATIONS OF THIS THERAPY?:
A. Impetigo
B. Conjunctivitis
C. Pustules
D. Pyarthrosis
E. Fatal sepsis and meningitis

Ref. Amer J Dis Child
123:45, January, 1972

SYPHILIS AND SEROLOGY

426. FALSE-POSITIVE REACTIONS FOR SYPHILIS (VDRL) MAY BE CLASSIFIED AS CHRONIC WHEN THEY PERSIST FOR SIX MONTHS OR LONGER. WHICH OF THE FOLLOWING ARE COMMONLY ASSOCIATED WITH TITERS OF 1:1 TO 1:4 FOR THIS PERIOD OF TIME?:
A. Smallpox vaccination
B. Narcotic addicts
C. Atypical pneumonia
D. Systemic lupus erythematosus
E. Infectious mononucleosis

Ref. N Engl J Med
284:642, March 25, 1971

TOXOCARIASIS

427. THE DIAGNOSIS OF TOXOCARIASIS IN CHILDREN IS BEST SUPPORTED IN THE LABORATORY BY WHICH OF THE FOLLOWING?:
A. Complement fixation test
B. Fluorescent antibody test
C. Muscle biopsy
D. Standardized skin test with toxocara antigen
E. Stool examination for ova

Ref. Br Med J
3:663, September 19, 1970

428. TOXOCARIASIS IN CHILDREN HAS BEEN ASSOCIATED WITH WHICH OF THE FOLLOWING CLINICAL SYNDROMES?:
A. Hepatomegaly with eosinophilia
B. Myocarditis
C. Endophthalmitis
D. Asthma or pneumonitis
E. Seizures

Ref. Br Med J 3:663, September 19, 1970

ANTIBIOTICS

FOR THE FOLLOWING MATCHING QUESTIONS CHOOSE THE ONE STATEMENT IN THE RIGHT HAND COLUMN WHICH BEST APPLIES TO THE STATEMENT IN THE LEFT HAND COLUMN. STATEMENTS ON THE RIGHT MAY BE USED MORE THAN ONCE:

INFECTING ORGANISM	DRUG OF FIRST CHOICE
429. ___ Salmonella typhi	A. Tetracycline
430. ___ Rocky Mountain spotted fever	B. Amphotericin B
431. ___ Vaccinia	C. Griseofulvin
432. ___ Candida albicans	D. Chloramphenicol
433. ___ Histoplasma capsulatum	E. Methisazone

Ref. Med Lett Drugs Ther Page 7, January, 1971

INFECTING ORGANISM	DRUG OF FIRST CHOICE
434. ___ Neisseria meningitidis	A. Ampicillin
435. ___ Klebsiella pneumoniae	B. Chloramphenicol
436. ___ Listeria monocytogenes	C. Erythromycin
437. ___ Proteus mirabilis	D. Gentamicin
438. ___ Shigella	E. Penicillin G

Ref. Med Lett Drugs Ther Page 7, January, 1971

ANTIBIOTICS

FOR THE FOLLOWING MATCHING QUESTIONS CHOOSE THE ONE STATEMENT IN THE RIGHT HAND COLUMN WHICH BEST APPLIES TO THE STATEMENT IN THE LEFT HAND COLUMN. STATEMENTS ON THE RIGHT MAY BE USED MORE THAN ONCE:

INFECTING ORGANISM	DRUG OF FIRST CHOICE
439. ___ Corynebacterium diphtheriae	A. Erythromycin
440. ___ Clostridium tetani	B. Penicillin G
441. ___ Enterobacter (Aerobacter)	C. Gentamicin
442. ___ Bacteroides	D. Ampicillin
443. ___ Mycoplasma pneumoniae	E. Tetracycline

Ref. Med Lett Drugs Ther Page 7, January, 1971

PARASITIC INFECTIONS

INFECTING ORGANISM	DRUG OF FIRST CHOICE
444. ___ Ascaris lumbricoides	A. Bephenium
445. ___ Trichuris trichiura (whipworm)	B. Piperazine citrate
446. ___ Visceral larva migrans	C. Thiabendazole
447. ___ Trichinella spiralis (trichinosis)	D. Hexylresorcinol
448. ___ Ancylostoma duodenale (hookworm)	E. No specific therapy

Ref. Med Lett Drugs Ther
Page 23, January, 1971

ANTIBIOTIC DOSAGE AND RENAL FUNCTION

EXCLUDING NEPHROTOXIC AGENTS, DRUG DOSAGE NEEDS LITTLE OR NO ADJUSTMENT IF CREATININE CLEARANCE IS ABOVE 25%. IN THE PRESENCE OF RENAL IMPAIRMENT, ANTIBIOTICS FALL INTO THREE CATEGORIES. MATCH THE FOLLOWING ANTIMICROBIALS:

A. Retained to a major degree
B. Moderately retained (intermediate)
C. Retained little or not at all

449. ___ Penicillins
450. ___ Neomycin
451. ___ Isoniazid
452. ___ Lincomycin
453. ___ Doxycycline
454. ___ Gentamicin
455. ___ Oxytetracycline
456. ___ Cephalosporins
457. ___ Polymyxins
458. ___ Erythromycin

Ref. Hospital Pract
7:41, January, 1972

CYTOMEGALOVIRUSES AND INFECTIOUS MONONUCLEOSIS

CYTOMEGALOVIRUSES HAVE BEEN RECENTLY SHOWN TO BE RESPONSIBLE FOR A SYNDROME WHICH CLOSELY MIMICS INFECTIOUS MONONUCLEOSIS. THIS MAY DEVELOP SPONTANEOUSLY OR IN PATIENTS PERFUSED WITH FRESH BLOOD IN CONNECTION WITH OPEN-HEART SURGERY.
MATCH THE FOLLOWING:

A. Cytomegalovirus infection
B. Infectious mononucleosis
C. Both
D. Neither

459. ___ Relative and absolute lymphocytosis
460. ___ Atypical lymphocytes
461. ___ Tonsillitis and lymphadenitis
462. ___ Abnormal liver-function tests
463. ___ Rubelliform rash
464. ___ Positive heterophile antibody test
465. ___ Myocarditis and electrocardiographic abnormalities
466. ___ Significant hepatosplenomegaly

Ref. J Infect Dis
123:555, May, 1971

FOR EACH OF THE FOLLOWING MULTIPLE CHOICE QUESTIONS, SELECT THE ONE APPROPRIATE ANSWER:

BENIGN PAROXYSMAL VERTIGO

467. BENIGN PAROXYSMAL VERTIGO OF CHILDHOOD IS CHARACTERIZED BY ALL OF THE FOLLOWING, EXCEPT:
A. Normal electroencephalograms
B. Nystagmus
C. Preservation of full awareness during and after an attack
D. Normal audiograms
E. Normal vestibular function during caloric testing

Ref. Neurology
20:1108, November, 1970

BRAIN SCANNING IN CHILDREN

468. BRAIN TUMORS ARE THE MOST COMMON SOLID TUMORS OF CHILDHOOD. EACH OF THE FOLLOWING IS CORRECT IN RESPECT TO THE USE OF TECHNETIUM-99m SCANS OF THE POSTERIOR FOSSA IN CHILDREN, EXCEPT:
A. The intensity of the uptake has no relationship to the relative malignancy of the underlying tumor
B. Factors contributing to the high degree of accuracy in the diagnosis of posterior fossa tumors in children include careful positioning
C. Technetium-99m does not cross the blood-brain barrier except as it has been disrupted by neoplasm, hemorrhage or inflammation
D. Medulloblastomas have rarely failed to visualize
E. Cystic cerebellar astrocytomas may be poorly visualized

Ref. Clin Pediatr
10:210, April, 1971

CEREBRORETINAL DEGENERATIONS

469. THE CEREBRORETINAL DEGENERATIONS ARE A GROUP OF HEREDITARY DISEASES WITH VARYING KNOWN AND UNKNOWN BIOCHEMICAL DEFECTS. RETINAL CHERRY-RED SPOTS ARE SEEN IN ALL OF THE FOLLOWING, EXCEPT:
A. Tay-Sachs
B. Niemann-Pick (Crocker's group C)
C. Generalized gangliosidosis
D. Infantile Gaucher's
E. Juvenile amaurotic idiocy (Spielmeyer-Vogt)

Ref. J Pediatr
79:183, August, 1971

CONVULSIONS, FEBRILE

470. IN THE MANAGEMENT OF FEBRILE CONVULSIONS IN CHILDREN ALL OF THE FOLLOWING ARE ACCEPTED AS CORRECT, EXCEPT:
A. Recurrence of febrile convulsions can be largely prevented by continuous prophylactic phenobarbital therapy
B. The majority of febrile seizures terminate spontaneously without specific therapy
C. Episodic phenobarbital prophylactic therapy appears effective in reducing the risk of a recurring febrile convulsion
D. It is not known whether or not recurrent febrile convulsions may predispose to epilepsy later in life for a small minority of children
E. Approximately 3 per cent of children experience a convulsion with fever in their first five years of life

Ref. J Pediatr
78:1083 June, 1971

DEPRIVATION, MATERNAL STUDY

471. THE LONG TERM PROGNOSIS FOR THE INFANT WHO FAILS TO THRIVE BECAUSE OF MATERNAL DEPRIVATION IS SUCH THAT A CLOSER STUDY OF THE MOTHER'S PERSONALITY STRUCTURE IS CRUCIAL TO INSURE PROPER MANAGEMENT. ALL OF THE FOLLOWING HAVE SUGGESTED THE PRESENCE OF A MATERNAL CHARACTER DISORDER, EXCEPT:

A. A limited capacity for concern
B. A limited ability to adapt to changes in the environment
C. A desire for an anaclitic relationship with an intense need to be taken care of
D. A response to a problem-solving, psychotherapeutic approach over many months
E. The use of denial, isolation and projection as major mechanisms of defense

Ref. J Pediatr 79:209, August, 1971

EPILEPSY, SUDDEN DEATH

472. UNEXPECTED SUDDEN DEATH OF EPILEPTICS WHICH IS UNRELATED TO STATUS EPILEPTICUS OR SUPERVENING ACCIDENTS OR CONCOMITANT DISEASE WAS FOUND IN A SERIES OF AUTOPSIES TO BE MOST OFTEN ASSOCIATED WITH:

A. Mechanical asphyxia
B. Aspiration of vomitus
C. Intracranial hemorrhage
D. Pulmonary edema
E. No satisfactory anatomic cause of death

Ref. Neurology 21:682, July, 1971

FACIAL PARALYSIS

473. IN A GROUP OF 61 CHILDREN WITH FACIAL PARALYSIS THE MOST COMMON ETIOLOGY IDENTIFIED WAS:

A. Birth trauma
B. Bell's palsy
C. Otitis media
D. Postimmunization
E. Viral diseases (varicella, mumps, herpes, etc.)

Ref. Pediatrics 49:102, 1972

HYPERKINESIS

474. THE "HYPERACTIVITY SYNDROME" OF CHILDHOOD APPEARS TO RESULT FROM AN INTERACTION OF MULTIPLE FACTORS, BOTH BIOLOGICAL AND ENVIRONMENTAL. WHICH OF THE FOLLOWING APPEARS TO BE THE MOST CRUCIAL IN PRODUCING HYPERKINESIS?:

A. Neurologic dysfunction
B. Mental subnormality
C. Family psychopathology
D. Abnormal electroencephalogram
E. Complications of pregnancy

Ref. J Pediatr 79:618, October, 1971

HYPERKINESIS AND DRUGS

475. OF THE NUMEROUS MEDICATIONS WHICH HAVE BEEN EMPLOYED IN THE TREATMENT OF HYPERKINETIC CHILDREN THE MOST COMMONLY PRESCRIBED IS:
A. Dexedrine
B. Ritalin
C. Mellaril
D. Atarax
E. Valium

Ref. Med Insight 3:22, November, 1971

HEADACHE AND PTOSIS

476. A 10 YEAR-OLD BOY WITH A HISTORY OF HEADACHE AND VOMITING OF 18 HOURS DURATION SUDDENLY DEVELOPS PTOSIS, DILATATION OF THE PUPIL AND INABILITY TO ADDUCT THE LEFT EYE. THERE IS COMPLETE RECOVERY IN TWO WEEKS. THE MOST LIKELY DIAGNOSIS IS:
A. Ophthalmoplegic migraine
B. Intracranial aneurysm
C. Myasthenia gravis
D. Intracranial tumor
E. Polyneuritis cranialis

Ref. Amer J Dis Child 122:237, September, 1971

NEUROBLASTOMA AND THE CNS

477. THE NATURAL HISTORY OF NEUROBLASTOMA HAS BEEN ASSOCIATED WITH ALL OF THE FOLLOWING CENTRAL NERVOUS SYSTEM MANIFESTATIONS, EXCEPT:
A. Hematogenous metastases to brain
B. Compression of the brain from skull metastasis
C. Opsoclonus
D. Differentiation into normal sympathetic nervous tissue
E. Ataxia

Ref. J Pediatr 75:987, December, 1969

DIAZEPAM

478. FEW DRUGS HAVE HAD SUCH WIDE CLINICAL USE IN SUCH A VARIETY OF CONDITION AS DIAZEPAM (VALIUM) EACH OF THE FOLLOWING STATEMENTS IS CORRECT IN REGARD TO THE USE OF DIAZEPAM, EXCEPT:
A. The drug has shown much promise in petit mal
B. Its parenteral use may be the method of choice in terminating status epilepticus
C. Parenteral administration of diazepam for status epilepticus requires observation for respiratory depression and hypotension
D. Diazepam has proved valuable in the treatment of tetanus, facial tics and phenothiazine-induced dyskinesia
E. There appears to be little tendency for seizures to recur after they have been controlled by the intravenous use of diazepam

Ref. Develop. Med Child Neurol 12:655, 1970
AMA Drug Evaluations 1:254, 1971

PLANTAR REFLEX OF THE NEWBORN

479. IN THE INTERPRETATION OF THE PLANTAR REFLEX IN THE NEWBORN ALL OF THE FOLLOWING ARE OBSERVED, EXCEPT:
A. The first movement of the great toe should always determine the response after the onset of stimulation
B. The plantar response may be influenced by the position of the infant's head
C. Most infants have a bilateral extensor response
D. Position of the foot at the onset of stimulation is critical to the type of response
E. The intensity of the stimulus, light or firm, greatly influences the type of reflex seen Ref. N Engl J Med 285:502, August 26, 1971

SUBACUTE SCLEROSING PANENCEPHALITIS

480. SUBACUTE SCLEROSING PANENCEPHALITIS OF DAWSON REPRESENTS ENDOGENOUS REINFECTION BY THE MEASLES VIRUS. EACH OF THE FOLLOWING STATEMENTS IS CORRECT, EXCEPT:
A. The latent period ranges from 2 to 17 years after the natural disease
B. The disease has been reported to have followed the administration of the live-virus vaccine
C. Measles virus has been seen in sections of brain tissue on electronmicroscopy
D. Measles virus has not been cultured from infected brain tissue
E. Extremely high levels of measles antibodies are present in the serum and spinal fluid Ref. N Engl J Med 284:769, April 8, 1971

TAY-SACHS DISEASE

481. THE FIRST MASS SCREENING PROGRAM TO DETECT CARRIERS OF TAY-SACHS DISEASE BEGAN IN 1971 IN THE BALTIMORE-WASHINGTON AREA. EACH OF THE FOLLOWING CHARACTERIZES TAY-SACHS DISEASE, EXCEPT:
A. One out of thirty Americans of Ashkenazi Jewish origin are carriers
B. The incidence of carriers in Sephardic Jews is many times greater than that of non-Jews
C. Amniocentesis can detect the absence of the enzyme, hexosaminidase, which results in Tay-Sachs disease
D. No effective therapy exists for Tay-Sachs disease
E. Parents of Tay-Sachs children show a 50 percent reduction in the enzyme, hexosaminidase Ref. JAMA 216:1097, May, 17, 1971

TETANUS

482. TETANUS IS A DISEASE IN WHICH THERE IS A SELECTIVE DEPRESSION OF INHIBITION IN THE CENTRAL NERVOUS SYSTEM. MANY OF THE NEUROLOGICAL SEQUELAE IN SURVIVORS SEEM TO BE SELF-LIMITING, AND HAVE INCLUDED ALL OF THE FOLLOWING, EXCEPT:
A. Fits and myoclonus
B. Abnormal electroencephalograms in about one-half
C. Postural hypotension
D. Hyposmia
E. Mild memory disturbance and irritability
Ref. Lancet Page 826, April 24, 1971

TUBEROUS SCLEROSIS AND SKIN LESIONS

483. IN AN INFANT WITH A SEIZURE DISORDER AND DEVELOPMENTAL RETARDATION, WHICH OF THE SKIN LESIONS WHICH ARE ASSOCIATED WITH TUBEROUS SCLEROSIS, WOULD BE FOUND MOST FREQUENTLY AT BIRTH?:

A. Café au lait spots
B. Shagreen patch
C. Macular leukoderma
D. Adenoma sebaceum
E. Poliosis

Ref. Amer J Dis Child 123:34, January, 1972

VENTRICULO-JUGULAR SHUNTS

484. CLOT FORMATION IN OR ABOUT THE DISTAL END OF THE VENTRICULO-JUGULAR SHUNT HAS BEEN A LEADING CAUSE OF SHUNT DYSFUNCTION AND ASCENDING INFECTION. IN A STUDY OF 30 CHILDREN WITH V-J SHUNTS ALL OF THE FOLLOWING WERE OBSERVED, EXCEPT:

A. High incidence of elevated titers of fibrin split products
B. Significant reductions in the lifespan of transfused platelets
C. Platelet aggregation at the catheter tip as a forerunner of thrombus formation
D. Increased platelet survival with the administration of aspirin and dipyridamole
E. High degree of thrombus prevention in areas of high flow with anticoagulants (heparin)

Ref. J Pediatr 80:21, January, 1972

FOR EACH OF THE FOLLOWING QUESTIONS, SELECT THE ONE APPROPRIATE ANSWER BY USING THE KEY OUTLINED BELOW:

1. If A, B and C are correct
2. If A and C are correct
3. If B and D are correct
4. If all are correct
5. If all are incorrect

ATAXIA

485. ACUTE ATAXIA IN CHILDREN HAS BEEN ASSOCIATED WITH WHICH OF THE FOLLOWING?:

A. Neuroblastoma
B. Postexanthematous encephalitis
C. Neurotropic viral encephalitis
D. Lead intoxication
E. Dilantin intoxication

Ref. Am J Dis Child 122:257, September, 1971

DYSAUTONOMIA, FAMILIAL

486. FAMILIAL DYSAUTONOMIA, A SYNDROME WHICH IS CHARACTERIZED BY AUTONOMIC-NERVOUS-SYSTEM DYSFUNCTION, IS ASSOCIATED WITH WHICH OF THE FOLLOWING?:

A. Occurs primarily in Ashkenazi Jewish children
B. Increased urinary excretion of homovanillic acid (HVA), a urinary metabolite of dopamine
C. Decreased urinary excretion of vanillymandelic acid (VMA)
D. Absence of the enzyme that converts dopamine to norepinephrine, dopamine-B-hydroxylase (DBH) in the plasma of many patients
E. Decreased DBH activity in the plasma of mothers of patients

Ref. N Engl J Med
285:938, October, 21, 1971

HEMOLYTIC-UREMIC SYNDROME

487. THE DIAGNOSIS OF HEMOLYTIC-UREMIC SYNDROME SHOULD BE CONSIDERED IN SEVERE ACUTE AND SUBACUTE ENCEPHALOPATHIES OF OBSCURE ORIGIN IN CHILDHOOD. WHICH OF THE FOLLOWING MAJOR NEUROLOGIC SIGNS HAVE BEEN SEEN IN MOST CHILDREN WITH THIS ASSOCIATION IN THIS SYNDROME?:

A. Decerebrate spasms
B. Convulsions
C. Aphasia or cortical blindness
D. Coma
E. Hemiparesis

Ref. Aust Pediatr J
7:28, 1971

HYDROCEPHALUS, NORMAL PRESSURE

488. NORMAL PRESSURE HYDROCEPHALUS IN CHILDREN IS CHARACTERIZED BY WHICH OF THE FOLLOWING?:

A. Symptoms which suggest brain stem or cortical injury
B. Progressive dilatation of the ventricles
C. Satisfactory response to shunting
D. Unusual persistance of residual air in ventricular system following contrast studies
E. Most common after posterior fossa surgery

Ref. Pediatrics
49:50, January, 1972

INTRACRANIAL ANTERIOVENOUS FISTULA IN INFANCY

489. INFANTS WITH AN INTRACRANIAL ARTERIOVENOUS FISTULA SHOW WHICH OF THE FOLLOWING?:

A. Wide arterial pulse pressure
B. Fall in pulmonary artery pressure after breathing 95% oxygen
C. Right ventricular hypertension
D. Low oxygen saturation in the right atrium
E. Accurate delineation of the defect for neurosurgical attack by left ventricular angiography

Ref. Pediatrics
49:30, January, 1972

490. AN INTRACRANIAL ARTERIOVENOUS FISTULA IN A NEWBORN INFANT SHOULD BE SUSPECTED WHEN WHICH OF THE FOLLOWING ARE NOTED IN COMBINATION?:

A. Cardiomegaly
B. Cranial bruit
C. Congestive heart failure in the first day of life
D. Hyperdynamic cardiac impulse
E. Good peripheral pulses

Ref. Pediatrics 49:30, January, 1972

PARAPLEGIA, TRAUMATIC IN INFANCY

491. AUTOMOBILE ACCIDENTS ARE THE MOST COMMON CAUSE OF INJURIES TO CHILDREN, AND TRAUMATIC PARAPLEGIA IS A TRAGEDY WHICH IS OFTEN PREVENTABLE. WHICH OF THE FOLLOWING ARE CORRECT?:

A. Massive and extensive softening of the spinal cord may follow compression of the anterior spinal artery without observable vessel thrombosis
B. Crying in response to a painful stimulus applied to the foot indicates always that the sensory pathway is intact
C. Infants may sustain extensive spinal cord injury without permanent radiological changes
D. Dislocation of the cervical spine in a child is not known to reduce spontaneously
E. The most secure location for an infant in an auto is in his mother's lap

Ref. JAMA 219:38, January 3, 1972

HEMATOMA, SUBDURAL OF INFANCY

492. THE PROGNOSIS IN SUBDURAL HEMATOMAS OF INFANCY DEPENDS LARGELY ON THE CONDITION OF THE BRAIN AT THE TIME OF TREATMENT. WHICH OF THE FOLLOWING STATEMENTS APPLIES TO THE DIAGNOSIS AND TREATMENT?:

A. An attempt should be made to aspirate subdural fluid during a diagnostic tap because of the viscosity of the collection
B. Transillumination is ineffective in the diagnosis of subdural hematomas
C. Craniotomy for the evacuation of the hematoma and stripping of the membranes is frequently necessary for cure
D. Examination of the eyegrounds does little to differentiate subdural hematoma from hydrocephalus
E. Subdural hematomas are rarely bilaterial, and symmetrical weakness of the extremities suggests another diagnosis

Ref. Clin Pediatr 10:597, October, 1971

SEIZURES AND ANTICONVULSANT THERAPY

493. THE PHYSICIAN SHOULD BE LOATH TO STOP ANTICONVULSANT THERAPY IN AN EPILEPTIC CHILD WITH A FOUR-YEAR REMISSION IF WHICH OF THE FOLLOWING ARE PRESENT?:

A. The seizures began after nine years of age
B. Continuation of seizures for more than six years before control with anticonvulsants
C. Seizures were Jacksonian or multiple in type
D. Presence of psychologic or neurologic deficits and the seizures began after the third year of life
E. Little change in the electroencephalogram despite the four-year period of seizure-free observation

Ref. N Engl J Med 286:169, January 27, 1972

SELF-MUTILATION

494. SELF-MUTILATION MAY BE AN ASSOCIATED FEATURE OF WHICH OF THE FOLLOWING ENTITIES?:
   A. de Lange syndrome
   B. Familial dysautonomia
   C. Lesch-Nyhan syndrome
   D. Trisomy 18
   E. XXY

Ref. J Pediatr 78:506, March, 1971

MYASTHENIA GRAVIS

ALTHOUGH MYASTHENIA GRAVIS IN THE NEWBORN INFANT IS NOT COMMON, IT HAS BECOME POSSIBLE TO CLASSIFY NEONATAL AND CONGENITAL FORMS OF THIS DISEASE.
MATCH THE FOLLOWING:

495. ___ Familial tendency
496. ___ Mother myasthenic
497. ___ Symptoms transient
498. ___ Symptoms mild
499. ___ Ptosis and ophthalmoplegia uncommon

A. Neonatal
B. Congenital
C. Both
D. Neither

Ref. Am J Dis Child 122:356, October, 1971

CEREBRORETINAL DEGENERATIONS

THE BEDSIDE DIAGNOSIS OF THE CEREBRORETINAL DEGENERATIONS IS AIDED BY CLASSIFYING THOSE CHILDREN WITH NEUROLOGICAL DEFICITS ACCORDING TO THE PRESENCE OR ABSENCE OF HEPATOSPLENOMEGALY.
MATCH THE FOLLOWING:

A. Without marked visceromegaly
B. With marked visceromegaly

500. ___ Infantile amaurotic idiocy (Tay-Sach's)
501. ___ Generalized gangliosidosis
502. ___ Infantile Gaucher's
503. ___ Juvenile amaurotic idiocy (Spielmeyer-Vogt)
504. ___ Niemann-Pick (Crocker's group C)

Ref. J Pediatr 79:183, August, 1971

FOR EACH OF THE FOLLOWING MULTIPLE CHOICE QUESTIONS, SELECT THE ONE APPROPRIATE ANSWER:

BLACK URINE

505. THE MOTHER OF A FOUR-YEAR OLD BOY REPORTS THAT HE HAS PASSED DARK URINE WHICH HAS BECOME BLACK ON STANDING. THERE IS A POSITIVE REACTION TO BENEDICT'S REAGENT. THE MOST LIKELY DIAGNOSIS IS:

A. Melanotic tumor
B. Phenol poisoning
C. Alcaptonuria
D. Homocystinuria
E. Indicanuria

Ref. Modern Medicine 39:110, June 28, 1971

AMNIOTIC FLUID AND AMINO ACIDS

506. THE FORMATION AND CIRCULATION OF AMNIOTIC FLUID REMAINS AN ENIGMA. INVESTIGATION INTO THE DIAGNOSTIC SIGNIFICANCE OF AMNIOTIC FLUID AMINO ACIDS HAS SUGGESTED ALL OF THE FOLLOWING, EXCEPT:

A. The maternal circulation and placenta can maintain a normal amino acid homeostasis in the fetus even if he is suffering from an inborn error of metabolism
B. The precursors to a metabolic block are readily metabolized and cleared by the mother, except as she is an obligate heterozygote for the disorder
C. Inheritable disorders of amino acid metabolism produce compounds that usually are readily metabolized by the mother
D. If the offending compound is nonmetabolizable it must be excreted by the maternal circulation, as is the case of a fetus with methylmalonic acidemia
E. Direct enzyme analyses from cultured amniotic fluid cells appear to be necessary for the diagnosis of most of the aminoacidopathies

Ref. Obstet Gynecol 37:550, April, 1971

BERIBERI, INFANTILE

507. SEVERAL THOUSAND DEATHS FROM INFANTILE BERIBERI ARE REPORTED ANNUALLY IN THE WORLD. MANY OF THESE CASES ARE SEEN IN BREAST-FED INFANTS WHEN THEIR MOTHER' S DIET CONSISTS ALMOST EXCLUSIVELY OF MILLED RICE. ALL OF THE FOLLOWING ARE CORRECT, EXCEPT:

A. The peak in infant mortality from this disease occurs between the second and the sixth month of life
B. Aphonia is seen often as a clinical manifestation of beriberi in infants
C. Gross edema is rare
D. Recovery may follow the injection of thiamine, often in a few hours
E. The child with beriberi is easily recognized, and his breast-feeding mother shares invariably in the clinical expression of thiamine deficiency

Ref. Clin Pediatr 10:250, May, 1971

BREAST MILK, BANKING

508. IN A REVIEW OF HUMAN MILK BANKING PRACTICES A NUMBER OF PROBLEMS IN REGARD TO COLLECTION, DECONTAMINATION, AND STORAGE HAVE BEEN IDENTIFIED. ALL OF THE FOLLOWING HAVE BEEN SUGGESTED AS CORRECT WITH THE EXCEPTION OF:

A. It is not necessary to monitor DDT concentration in the milk of individual donors
B. Regular surveillance of radioactive contaminants (Strontium-90, Iodine-131 and Cesium-137) in cow's milk indicates a relatively low level of radionuclides in the environment since the ban on atomic weapons testing in the atmosphere
C. Flash sterilization or classic pasteurization does not modify the immune substances in human milk
D. Frozen milk can be stored for extended periods with no appreciable change in composition
E. Environmental contaminants such as lead, arsenic and organophosphates present no problem since they are not transferred to milk in any appreciable quantities

Ref. Pediatrics
47:457, February, 1971

BREAST MILK AND DRUGS

509. AVAILABLE INFORMATION DERIVED FROM CLINICAL AND LABORATORY RESEARCH CONCERNING THE EXCRETION OF CHEMICALS AND DRUGS IN BREAST MILK IS SCANTY. ALL OF THE FOLLOWING DRUGS WHEN TAKEN IN THE USUAL DOSAGE APPEAR READILY IN BREAST MILK AND MAY POSE UNDESIRABLE PHARMOCOLOGIC EFFECTS ON THE INFANT, EXCEPT:

A. Chloramphenicol
B. Isoniazid
C. Progestin-estogen oral contraceptives
D. Caffeine
E. Reserpine

Ref. Nutrition Today
5:2, November 4, 1970

BREAST MILK AND JAUNDICE

510. PHYSIOLOGIC JAUNDICE OCCURS IN APPROXIMATELY 60 PER CENT OF ALL FULL TERM INFANTS AND TO AN EVEN GREATER EXTENT IN PREMATURES. BIOCHEMICALLY, THE ELEVATION IN SERUM BILIRUBIN RARELY EXCEEDS 15mgs. JAUNDICE IN NEWBORNS ASSOCIATED WITH BREAST MILK HAS BEEN ASSOCIATED WITH ALL OF THE FOLLOWING, EXCEPT:

A. Hyperbilirubinemia occurs in these infants as a result of inhibition of the hepatic microsomal enzyme-glucuronyl transferase
B. Approximately 1 per cent of breast-fed infants develop prolonged, unconjugated hyperbilirubinemia as the result of ingestion of pregnane-3 (alpha); 20 (beta) diol in the milk
C. Severe jaundice is usually not noted until the second week of life
D. Heat sterilization and boiling destroys and inactivates the inhibitory steroid
E. Kernicterus has not been described in breast milk associated jaundice which has been uncomplicated by hemolytic disease or other pathologic states

Ref. Pediatrics
47:456, February, 1971

FECAL FLORA OF BREAST-FED INFANTS

511. AN ENVIRONMENT OF LOW pH IN THE COLON OF BREAST-FED INFANTS APPEARS TO BE UNFAVORABLE FOR THE GROWTH OF GRAM-NEGATIVE ENTERIC ORGANISMS. THE PRODUCTION AND MAINTENANCE OF THIS ACID MEDIUM APPEARS TO BE INFLUENCED BY ALL OF THE FOLLOWING FACTORS, EXCEPT:
A. A lactobacillary flora
B. Intestinal contents which have an increased buffering capacity
C. A lower protein content of breast milk
D. A lower phosphate content of human milk
E. Increased lactose fermentation

Ref. Br Med J
3:338, August 7, 1971

CYTINOSIS

512. REFRACTORY RICKETS ASSOCIATED WITH MULTIPLE DEFECTS OF THE RENAL TUBULES IN A CHILD WITH PHOTOPHOBIA AND A CRAVING FOR MEAT SHOULD SUGGEST CYSTINOSIS. CYSTINE CRYSTALS ARE FOUND IN ALL OF THE FOLLOWING TISSUES, EXCEPT:
A. Bone marrow
B. Cornea
C. Rectal mucosa
D. Red blood cells
E. White blood cells

Ref. Pediatr Clin N Am
18:200, February, 1971

DE LANGE SYNDROME

513. BIOCHEMICAL AND GENETIC EVIDENCE SUGGESTS THAT THE DE LANGE SYNDROME MAY BE THE RESULT OF AN INHERITED METABOLIC ERROR. THE EXACT NATURE OF THE ENZYMATIC DEFECT IS UNCERTAIN. HOWEVER, RECENT STUDIES HAVE SHOWN ALL OF THE FOLLOWING BIOCHEMICAL FEATURES IN THE DE LANGE SYNDROME, EXCEPT:
A. Increased glutamic acid levels
B. Generalized hypoaminoaciduria
C. Elevated SGOT and SGPT levels
D. Hypogammaglobulinemia with normal levels of IgA, IgG and IgM
E. Increased serum alpha-ketoglutarate

Ref. Amer J Dis Child
121:401, May, 1971

GALACTOSEMIA, NEW FORM

514. A RECENTLY DISCOVERED VARIATION OF GALACTOSEMIA INVOLVING GALACTOKINASE DEFICIENCY HAS BEEN ASSOCIATED WITH BUT ONE OF THE FOLLOWING:
A. Hepatomegaly
B. Neonatal sepsis
C. Juvenile cataracts
D. Jaundice
E. Cirrhosis

Ref. N Engl J Med
284:753, April 8, 1971

HUNTER'S SYNDROME

515. IN AN IMPORTANT STUDY WHICH HAS IMPLICATIONS FOR THERAPEUTIC ATTEMPTS IN THE TREATMENT OF HEREDITARY DISEASES, DRAMATIC BIOCHEMICAL AND CLINICAL CHANGES IN TYPE II MUCOPOLYSACCHARIDOSIS (HUNTER'S SYNDROME) HAVE BEEN REPORTED WITH:

A. Anti-lymphocyte serum
B. Enzyme inductions
C. Transfusions of normal human leukocytes
D. Bone marrow transplantation
E. Exchange transfusion

Ref. Proc. Nat Acad Sci USA 68:1738, August, 1971

HYPOGLYCEMIA, NEONATAL

516. NEONATAL HYPOGLYCEMIA MAY RESULT FROM A WIDE VARIETY OF FACTORS AND A CORRECT DIAGNOSIS IS ESSENTIAL FOR PROPER MANAGEMENT. ALL OF THE FOLLOWING ARE CORRECT IN REGARD TO THIS METABOLIC DISTURBANCE IN THE NEWBORN, EXCEPT:

A. Serum values for glucose are approximately 10 to 15 per cent higher than those of whole blood
B. Most if not all infants with blood glucose values under 20 mgm per cent are symptomatic
C. Some symptomatic hypoglycemia in infants of diabetic mothers appears to be reactive to the vigorous and episodic administration of glucose resulting in increased insulin release
D. "Early" feeding and careful temperature regulation have decreased the incidence of symptomatic hypoglycemia in low-birth weight infants
E. Symptomatic hypoglycemia is rare with blood glucose values greater than 20 mgm per cent

Ref. J Pediatr 79:314, August, 1971

517. NEWER STUDIES IN THE EMERGENCY TREATMENT OF SYMPTOMATIC HYPOGLYCEMIA IN NEWBORN INFANTS HAVE SHOWN THE MOST IMPORTANT THERAPEUTIC MEASURE TO BE:

A. Glucagon
B. Intravenous hypertonic glucose
C. Prednisone
D. Intravenous fructose
E. Intravenous hypertonic galactose

Ref. J Pediatr 79:314, August, 1971

HYPOGLYCEMIA, SYMPTOMATIC

518. SYMPTOMATIC HYPOGLYCEMIA IS LEAST LIKELY TO BE MANIFEST IN WHICH OF THE FOLLOWING CONDITIONS?:

A. Infants of diabetic mothers
B. Fructosemia
C. Galactosemia
D. Islet cell tumor of pancreas
E. Leucine sensitivity

Ref. Br Med J 1:5, 1972

HYPOPROTEINEMIA IN TURNER OR NOONAN SYNDROME

519. HYPOPROTEINEMIA WITH NORMAL HEPATIC AND RENAL FUNCTION IN A CHILD WITH EITHER TURNER OR NOONAN SYNDROME SHOULD SUGGEST THE POSSIBILITY OF:
A. Congenital analbuminemia
B. Cystic fibrosis
C. Gluten-induced enteropathy
D. Intestinal lymphangiectasis
E. Leukemia

Ref. J Pediatr 80:269, February, 1972

INSULIN, FETAL RESPONSE

520. ALTHOUGH LITTLE IS KNOWN OF THE DEVELOPMENT OF INSULIN RESPONSE OF THE FETUS, ALL OF THE FOLLOWING ARE RECOGNIZED, EXCEPT:
A. The fetus has no significant plasma insulin response to the insulinogenic stimulus of maternally infused arginine
B. The newborn infant responds significantly to intravenous arginine infusion
C. The human placenta is permeable to insulin
D. Early in pregnancy fetal insulin response to sustained maternal hyperglycemia is negligible
E. The newborn responds to prolonged hyperglycemia with an elevation of plasma insulin

Ref. N Engl J Med 285:607, September 9, 1971

KETONURIA, NEONATAL

KETONURIA IN THE NEONATE SHOULD ALERT THE CLINICIAN TO UNUSUAL METABOLIC ABNORMALITIES. MATCH THE FOLLOWING CLINICAL AND BIOCHEMICAL FEATURES WITH THE PROPER SYNDROMES:
A. Growth delay, questionable mental retardation, marked hepatomegaly, hypoglycemia, increased plasma lactate, increased uric acid
B. Growth delay, mental retardation, hepatomegaly, hypoglycemia, neutropenia, thrombocytopenia, osteoporosis and elevated plasma glycine
C. Elevated blood glucose, elevated plasma lactate and uric acid
D. Growth delay, mental retardation, hypoglycemia, neutropenia, thrombocytopenia, osteoporosis, and elevated plasma glycine
E. Hepatomegaly, hypoglycemia, elevated plasma lactate and elevated uric acid

521. ___ Glycogen storage disease (type I)
522. ___ Diabetes mellitus, transient or permanent
523. ___ Fructose-1, 6 diphosphate deficiency
524. ___ Glycinemia (ketotic)
525. ___ Methylmalonic acidemia

Ref. J Pediatr 79:417, September, 1971

SELECT THE ONE APPROPRIATE ANSWER:

METABOLIC SCREENING

526. EXAMINATION OF THE URINE FOR CRYSTALS MAY BE A CLUE TO THE PRESENCE OF METABOLIC DISEASE. EACH OF THE FOLLOWING DISEASES MAY BE SUGGESTED BY URINE CRYSTALS, EXCEPT:

A. Cystinosis
B. Maple syrup urine disease
C. Orotic aciduria
D. Xanthinuria
E. Tyrosinemia

Ref. Pediatr Clin N Am 18:200, February, 1971

METABOLIC SCREENING

527. MENTAL RETARDATION, FAILURE TO THRIVE, UNEXPLAINED HEPATOMEGALY, OPHTHALMOLOGIC ABNORMALITIES (CATARACT, CORNEAL OPACITIES, SUBLUXATION OF THE LENS) AND NEUROLOGIC DISORDERS SHOULD SUGGEST THE NEED FOR METABOLIC SCREENING OF CHILDREN. A POSITIVE FERRIC CHLORIDE TEST ON URINE IS ASSOCIATED WITH ALL OF THE FOLLOWING METABOLIC DISEASES, EXCEPT:

A. Phenylketonuria
B. Tyrosinemia
C. Maple syrup urine disease
D. Histidinemia
E. Galactosemia

Ref. Pediatr Clin N Am 18:201, February, 1971

METABOLIC ODORS

528. THE CLINICIAN WITH A KEEN NOSE COULD RIGHTFULLY SUSPECT ALL BUT ONE OF THE FOLLOWING CONDITIONS AT THE BEDSIDE:

A. Phenylketonuria
B. Isovaleric acidemia
C. Defective oxidative decarboxylation of the branched chain amino acids
D. Methionine malabsorption syndrome
E. Homocystinuria

Ref. Pediatrics 41:993, May, 1968

MUCOPOLYSACCHARIDOSES

529. PATIENTS WITH ABNORMAL MUCOPOLYSACCHARIDE METABOLISM HAVE VARYING DEGREES OF SKELETAL, SOFT TISSUE AND SPECIFIC ORGAN INVOLVEMENT WHICH ACCOMPANY THE BIOCHEMICAL ERROR. EACH OF THE FOLLOWING HAS CORNEAL CLOUDING OF VARYING SEVERITY, EXCEPT:

A. Hurler
B. Hunter
C. Morquio
D. Scheie
E. Maroteaux-Lamy

Ref. J Pediatr 77:253, August, 1970

OBESITY AND THERAPEUTIC STARVATION

530. THERAPEUTIC STARVATION AS A MODE OF THERAPY FOR THE OBESE PATIENT HAS LED TO ALL OF THE FOLLOWING OBSERVATIONS, EXCEPT:

A. Increased urinary potassium excretion is observed from the utilization of lean body mass for gluconeogenesis
B. In fasting subjects, after the cessation of bowel evacuation, the kidneys become the sole, major excretory organ
C. The renal leak of electrolytes in therapeutic starvation may lead to hyponatraemic shock
D. The origin of urinary sodium loss appears to be from the breakdown of adipose tissue
E. A fall in blood pressure accompanies a prolonged fast

Ref. Br Med J
2:22, April 3, 1971

PKU AND THE EFFECTS OF DIET

531. THE WIDE VARIABILITY IN THE BIOCHEMICAL AND CLINICAL EXPRESSION OF PHENYLKETONURIA MAKES THE ASSESSMENT OF TREATMENT DIFFICULT. EACH OF THE FOLLOWING IS CORRECT IN PKU, EXCEPT:

A. PKU children has shown a slower rate of grow th on a diet of phenylalanine restriction
B. Electroencephalogram abnormalities in children placed on treatment in the newborn period are rare
C. The incidence of EEG abnormalities in late-treated patients is nearly that of untreated children
D. The incidence of seizures is the same in the treated and untreated groups
E. The younger the child at the time of initial dietary restriction, the more depressed are the effects on growth

Ref. Develop Med Child Neurol
13:63, 1971

SCURVY

532. TRITIUM-LABELED AND C-LABELED ASCORBIC ACID HAS LED TO MORE PRECISE KNOWLEDGE OF THE METABOLISM OF VITAMIN C. THE FIRST CLINICAL SIGN OF SCURVY TO APPEAR IN ADULT VOLUNTEERS WAS:

A. Hyperkeratosis
B. Coiled hairs
C. Gum changes
D. Arthralgia
E. Petechiae

Ref. Am J Clin Nutr
24:432, April, 1971

SJÖGRENS SYNDROME

533. MANY OF THE CLINICAL FEATURES OF SJÖGREN'S (SICCA) SYNDROME SUCH AS ICHTHYOSIS, KERATOCONJUNCTIVITIS, SALIVARY GLAND ENLARGEMENT AND DRYNESS OF THE EYES HAVE BEEN PRODUCED EXPERIMENTALLY IN HUMANS WITH DIETS WHICH HAVE BEEN DEFICIENT IN WHICH OF THE FOLLOWING?:

A. Vitamin A
B. Ascorbic acid
C. Pantothenic acid
D. Niacin
E. Vitamin E

Ref. Am J Clin Nutr 24:432, April, 1971

SWEAT CHLORIDES

534. ALTHOUGH NOT A SPECIFIC LABORATORY TEST, AN ELEVATED SWEAT CHLORIDE LEVEL IS THE MOST RELIABLE FINDING IN CYSTIC FIBROSIS. WHICH OF THE FOLLOWING HAS BEEN ASSOCIATED WITH INCREASED SWEAT CHLORIDES?:

A. Fucosidosis
B. Congenital adrenal hyperplasia with salt depletion
C. Malnourished children
D. Pitressin resistant diabetes insipidus
E. All of the above

Ref. Clin Pediatr 10:285, 1971

SWEAT CHLORIDES AND MINERALOCORTICOIDS

535. IN CHILDREN WITH MARGINAL ELEVATIONS OF SWEAT CHLORIDES THE EFFECT ON SWEAT ELECTROLYTES AFTER THE ADMINISTRATION OF A MINERALOCORTICOID HAS BEEN SUGGESTED AS A MEANS OF DIFFERENTIATING THE CHILD WITH CYSTIC FIBROSIS FROM THE NORMAL. EACH OF THE FOLLOWING OBSERVATIONS IS CORRECT, EXCEPT:

A. Mineralocorticoids do not significantly decrease the sodium content of sweat in patients with cystic fibrosis
B. Mineralocorticoids may decrease the sodium content of sweat in normal children
C. The corresponding rise in sweat potassium after mineralocorticoids in normal subjects is variable and at times absent
D. In patient's with cystic fibrosis adrenal function is normal
E. The sweating rate of children with cystic fibrosis is normal or close to normal

Ref. J Pediatr 78:1036, June, 1971

WILSON'S DISEASE

536. DELAY IN THE DIAGNOSIS OF WILSON'S DISEASE MAY ARISE BECAUSE OF THE VARIED MODES OF PRESENTATION. EACH OF THE FOLLOWING IS CORRECT, EXCEPT:

A. Hepatic involvement may precede the neurologic manifestations by several years
B. The liver disease is characterized clinically by features indistinguishable from acute infectious hepatitis
C. Isolated splenomegaly may be the earliest physical finding
D. The absence of Kayser-Fleischer rings excludes the diagnosis of Wilson's disease
E. The patient with Wilson's disease who bleeds from esophageal varices in unlikely to have prolonged survival

Ref. J Pediatr 78:578, April, 1971

537. INCREASED AWARENESS OF WILSON'S DISEASE IN THE PEDIATRIC POPULATION AND EARLIER DIAGNOSIS SHOULD IMPROVE THE PROGNOSIS OF THIS SERIOUS BUT TREATABLE INBORN ERROR OF METABOLISM. EACH OF THE FOLLOWING IS CORRECT, EXCEPT:

A. A normal level of serum ceruloplasmin excludes the diagnosis of Wilson's disease
B. The most informative laboratory finding is a quantitative increase in hepatic copper
C. Total serum copper concentrations may be low or normal and are not recommended as a diagnostic test
D. Quantitative analysis of the 24 hr. urinary excretion of copper in the absence of biliary obstruction may offer presumptive evidence of Wilson's disease
E. Treatment with d-penicillamine is a well established and accepted form of therapy

Ref. J Pediatr 78:578, April, 1971

FOR EACH OF THE FOLLOWING QUESTIONS, SELECT THE ONE APPROPRIATE ANSWER BY USING THE KEY OUTLINED BELOW:

1. If A, B and C are correct
2. If A and C are correct
3. If B and D are correct
4. If all are correct
5. If all are incorrect

CARBOHYDRATE INTOLERANCE

538. DISTURBANCES IN CARBOHYDRATE METABOLISM OCCUR FREQUENTLY IN ASSOCIATION WITH:

A. Acromegaly
B. Cushing's syndrome
C. Obesity
D. Pinealoma
E. Craniopharyngioma

Ref. J Pediatr 75:349, September, 1969

FEEDING, EARLY OF LOW BIRTH INFANTS

539. APPROPRIATE AND EARLY FEEDING OF THE LOW-BIRTH WEIGHT INFANT MINIMIZES WHICH OF THE FOLLOWING?:

A. Hyperbilirubinemia
B. Hypoglycemia
C. Increases in serum osmolality
D. Hypocalcemia
E. Hyperaminoacidemia

Ref. J Pediatr 79:694, October, 1971

GALACTOSEMIA, "CLASSIC"

540. "CLASSIC" GALACTOSEMIA DUE TO DEFICIENT GALACTOSE-1-PHOSPHATE URIDYLTRANSFERASE ACTIVITY HAS BEEN ASSOCIATED WITH WHICH OF THE FOLLOWING SYMPTOMS?:

A. Hepatomegaly
B. Neonatal sepsis
C. Cataracts
D. Jaundice
E. Failure to thrive

Ref. N Engl J Med 14:285, April 8, 1971

MATERNAL HYPERPHENYLALANINEMIA

541. FOUR CHILDREN WHO WERE BORN TO A MENTALLY NORMAL HYPERPHENYLALANINEMIC MOTHER WHOSE PLASMA PHENYLALININE LEVEL AVERAGED 16 mg/100 ml DEMONSTRATED WHICH OF THE FOLLOWING FINDINGS?:
A. Educable retarded children
B. Growth retardation
C. Minor congenital abnormalities which were not the same in all the children
D. Microcephaly
E. Unusual personality patterns

Ref. Pediatrics
48:401, September, 1971

HYPOGLYCEMIA, KETOTIC

542. WHICH OF THE FOLLOWING ARE CORRECT IN KETOTIC HYPOGLYCEMIA OF CHILDHOOD?:
A. More common in boys than girls
B. Often in children who were small for dates
C. Rarely presents in first year of life
D. Acetonuria an essential feature
E. Has been associated with cataract formation

Ref. Br Med J
1:5, January 1, 1972

INTRAVENOUS ALIMENTATION

543. TOTAL PARENTERAL ALIMENTATION IN NEWBORN AND YOUNG INFANTS HAS BEEN ASSOCIATED WITH WHICH OF THE FOLLOWING BIOCHEMICAL ABERRATIONS?:
A. Hyperammonemia
B. Hyperaminoacidemia
C. Metabolic acidosis
D. Elevated blood urea nitrogen
E. Elevations of liver enzymes (SGOT, SGPT)

Ref. Pediatrics
48:955, December, 1971

MARFAN'S SYNDROME AND HOMOCYSTINURIA

544. THE PATIENT DESCRIBED ORIGINALLY BY MARFAN IN 1896, IN ALL LIKELIHOOD, HAD HOMOCYSTINURIA. WHICH OF THE FOLLOWING, WHEN PRESENT, SERVE TO DIFFERENTIATE HOMOCYSTINURIA FROM MARFAN'S SYNDROME?:
A. Ectopia lentis
B. Severe psychomotor retardation
C. Dolichostenomely
D. Joint contractures
E. Cardiovascular anomalies

Ref. J Pediatr
79:717, October, 1971

PHENYLKETONURIA, MATERNAL

545. CHILDREN BORN OF MOTHERS WITH PHENYLKETONURIA HAVE SHOWN WHICH OF THE FOLLOWING ASSOCIATIONS?:
A. Microcephaly
B. Intra-uterine growth retardation
C. Mental retardation
D. Atypical phenylketonuria
E. Congenital heart disease

Ref. Lancet
1:210, January 31, 1970

PHENYLKETONURIA

546. RECOMMENDATIONS IN THE MANAGEMENT OF PKU HAVE INCLUDED WHICH OF THE FOLLOWING?:
A. Critical phenylalanine levels for the diagnosis of PKU have not been established
B. Reliance on the demonstration of urinary metabolites of phenylalanine by $FeCL_3$ or buffered iron salt stick tests alone as an indicator of dietary control are quite satisfactory
C. Precise therapeutic levels of phenylalanine have not been accurately defined
D. Confirmatory tests after a presumptive diagnosis of PKU need involve only phenylalanine levels
E. Intellectual impairment may be associated with the heterozygote whose fasting phenylalanine levels may be 1.5 to 2.5 times normal

Ref. Clin Pediatr
10:295, September, 1971

VITAMIN C

547. GREAT QUANTITIES OF VITAMIN C ARE BEING CONSUMED TO PREVENT AND TREAT THE COMMON COLD. WHICH OF THE FOLLOWING ARE REAL OR THEORETICAL SIDE EFFECTS FROM THE EXCESSIVE INGESTION OF VITAMIN C?:
A. Increased tendency to renal calculi in individuals with increased excretion of cystine
B. Increase in excretion of oxalic acid and possibility of urinary calculi
C. Reversal of anticoagulant activity of warfarin
D. Precipitation of crises in sickle cell disease
E. Potential for renal stones in individuals with a tendency to gout (urate stores)

Ref. Newsletter
Am Acad Pediatr
22:2, November 1, 1971

TRIGLYCERIDES, MEDIUM-CHAIN

548. WHICH OF THE FOLLOWING METABOLIC EFFECTS HAVE BEEN NOTED IN CHILDREN RECEIVING MEDIUM-CHAIN TRIGLYCERIDES?:
A. Somnolence in cirrhotic patients with hypoalbuminemia
B. Increase in fecal water loss
C. Exaggeration of ketosis in certain diabetics
D. Increase in the incidence of peptic ulcer since the intestinal absorption of fat aids in controlling gastric hydrogen ion secretions
E. Increase in fecal sodium and potassium excretion

Ref. DM
July, 1971

VITAMIN K

549. THE AMERICAN ACADEMY OF PEDIATRICS' COMMITTEE ON NUTRITION HAS SUGGESTED SUPPLEMENTATION OF THE DIET OF INFANTS WITH VITAMIN K IN WHICH OF THE FOLLOWING CLINICAL SITUATIONS?:
A. Infants on a meat base formula
B. Infants drinking a casein hydrolysate formula
C. Biliary atresia
D. Cystic fibrosis of the pancreas
E. Prolonged parenteral feeding or diarrhea

Ref. Pediatrics
48:483, September, 1971

HYPOGLYCEMIA, NEONATAL

MATCH THE FOLLOWING:

A. Neonatal hypoglycemia due to excessive insulin secretion
B. Neonatal hypoglycemia due to diminished liver and muscle glycogen in the presence of an increased oxygen consumption and metabolic rate
C. Both of the above
D. Neither of the above

550. ___ Glycogen storage disease, type 1
551. ___ Infants of toxemic mothers
552. ___ Infants of gestational diabetic mothers
553. ___ Severe erythroblastosis fetalis
554. ___ "Small-for-dates" infants

Ref. J Pediatr
79:314, August, 1971

MALNUTRITION, PROTEIN-CALORIE

PROTEIN-CALORIE MALNUTRITION IN YOUNG CHILDREN REPRESENTS THE MOST IMPORTANT AND WIDESPREAD NUTRITIONAL PROBLEM IN THE WORLD. THE TWO MAJOR CLINICAL EXPRESSIONS ARE KWASHIORKOR AND NUTRITIONAL MARASMUS. WHICH OF THE FOLLOWING CLINICAL FEATURES IS MORE TYPICAL OF:

A. Kwashiorkor
B. Marasmus
C. Both
D. Neither

555. ___ Edema
556. ___ Anemia
557. ___ Hair changes
558. ___ Hepatomegaly
559. ___ Mental changes
560. ___ Growth failure
561. ___ Preservation of appetite
562. ___ Dermatosis (flaky paint)

Ref. Scope Manual on Nutrition
Page 35, 1970

TRIGLYCERIDES, MEDIUM-CHAIN

THE EFFICACY OF MEDIUM-CHAIN TRIGLYCERIDES IN REDUCING STEATORRHEA IN CHILDREN HAS BEEN DEMONSTRATED IN WHICH OF THE FOLLOWING MALABSORPTIVE DISORDERS?:

A. MCT of considerable therapeutic value
B. MCT helpful as adjunct to therapy
C. MCT rarely necessary

563. ___ Massive bowel resection
564. ___ Intestinal lymphangiectasia
565. ___ Ileal disease with steatorrhea
566. ___ A-beta lipoproteinemia with steatorrhea
567. ___ Pancreatic insufficiency
568. ___ Blind-loop syndrome responsive to antibiotics
569. ___ Biliary atresia
570. ___ Tropical and nontropical sprue
571. ___ Blind-loop syndrome unresponsive to antibiotics
572. ___ Regional enteritis with steatorrhea

Ref. J Pediatr
79:383, September, 1971
DM July, 1971

HYPERLIPOPROTEINEMIAS, FAMILIAL

THE PREVENTION OF ATHEROSCLEROSIS UNDOUBTEDLY INVOLVES THE PEDIATRICIAN WHO SHOULD FAMILIARIZE HIMSELF WITH THE FAMILIAL HYPERLIPOPROTEINEMIAS. BY MEANS OF ELECTROPHORESIS OR ANALYTICAL ULTRACENTRIFUGATION, LIPOPROTEINS CAN BE SEPARATED. MATCH THE CLINICAL DESCRIPTIONS WITH THE CLASSIFICATIONS OF HYPERLIPOPROTEINEMIA:

A. Type I, exogenous hyperlipidemia, Buerger-Grutz disease, autosomal recessive, rare
B. Type II, essential familial hypercholesterolemia, simple mendelian dominant, common
C. Type III, idiopathic hyperlipidemia, recessive (?), less common than II or IV
D. Type IV, endogenous hyperlipidemia, most common, simple mendelian dominant (?)
E. Type V, mixed hyperlipidemia, probably genetic variant of type IV, rare

573. ___ Onset in childhood or adulthood, xanthelasma, xanthoma of finger creases, arcus cornea, accelerated atherosclerosis, cholesterol markedly increased, glucose tolerance usually normal, secondary forms with nephrotic syndrome, hypothyroidism and liver disease

574. ___ Onset in adulthood, xanthelasma, eruptive xanthomas, triglycerides markedly increased, abnormal glucose tolerance, secondary forms with glycogen storage disease, diabetes mellitus, hypothyroidism

575. ___ Onset in childhood, hepatosplenomegaly, lipemia retinalis, low incidence of cardiovascular disease, normal glucose tolerance, eruptive xanthomas and triglycerides markedly increased. Secondary forms seen in systemic lupus erythematosus and lymphoma

576. ___ Onset in adulthood, hepatosplenomegaly, infrequent cardiovascular disease, triglycerides increased, glucose tolerance abnormal, eruptive xanthomas, obesity, secondary forms in insulin dependent diabetes mellitus, pancreatitis and alcoholism

577. ___ Onset in adulthood, high incidence of cardiovascular disease, palmar xanthomas, abnormal glucose tolerance, cholesterol and triglycerides both increased

Ref. Modern Med
Page 97, April 5, 1971

FOR EACH OF THE FOLLOWING MULTIPLE CHOICE QUESTIONS, SELECT THE ONE APPROPRIATE ANSWER:

RETROLENTAL FIBROPLASIA

578. THE CURRENT TREND OF USING HIGH OXYGEN CONCENTRATIONS IN THE MANAGEMENT OF THE RESPIRATORY DISTRESS SYNDROME SHOULD ALERT PEDIATRICIANS TO THE POTENTIAL FOR INCREASING THE INCIDENCE OF RETROLENTAL FIBROPLASIA. EACH OF THE FOLLOWING IS CORRECT, EXCEPT:
A. At the present time there are no data to define the tolerance of the retina to various Po_2 levels by duration of administration of oxygen or the age of the infant
B. Vasoconstriction is the initial clinical manifestation of oxygen toxicity on the retinal vasculature
C. There is no effective treatment for retrolental fibroplasia
D. Signs of the active phase of retrolental fibroplasia generally appear after the infant has been removed from oxygen
E. Documented retrolental fibroplasia has not been reported in full-term infants or in premature infants not receiving oxygen

Ref. Pediatr Clin N Am
17: May, 1970

FLUORESCEIN AND REACTIONS

579. THE MOST COMMON REACTION TO THE USE OF INTRAVENOUS FLUORESCEIN IN DIAGNOSTIC OPHTHALMOLOGY HAS BEEN:
A. Cardiac arrest
B. Urticaria
C. Hypotension
D. Hemolysis of red cells
E. Hematuria

Ref. Am J Ophthamol
72:865, November, 1971

PHOTOPHOBIA

580. PHOTOPHOBIA IS ASSOCIATED WITH ALL OF THE FOLLOWING SYSTEMIC DISEASES, EXCEPT:
A. Chediak-Higashi syndrome
B. Familial dysautonomia
C. Cystinosis
D. Acrodynia
E. Hartnup disease

Ref. DM
February, 1971

CHRONIC IRIDOCYCLITIS

581. CHRONIC IRIDOCYCLITIS IS UNUSUAL IN CHILDREN BUT IS MOST OFTEN FOUND IN ASSOCIATION WITH JUVENILE RHEUMATOID ARTHRITIS. EACH OF THE FOLLOWING STATEMENTS IS CORRECT, EXCEPT:
A. The children at greatest risk for developing iridocyclitis have a monoarticular onset or oligoarthritic course of their disease
B. The earliest manifestations of iridocyclitis can be detected only by slit lamp examination
C. Iridocyclitis may precede the onset of arthritis or appear when the arthritis is inactive
D. Iridocyclitis responds promptly to steroids
E. There is less urgency for routine screening for silent iridocyclitis when juvenile rheumatoid arthritis patients reach adulthood

Ref. Arthritis Rheum
13:406, July, August, 1970

RETINOPATHY, CHARACTERISTIC

582. A 16 YEAR-OLD CHILD WITH REDUCED VISION WHO DEMONSTATES ON OPHTHALMOSCOPIC EXAMINATION TINY GLISTENING CRYSTALS IN THE SMALL VESSELS ABOUT THE MACULA SHOULD BE SUSPECTED OF:
A. Cystinosis
B. Wilson's disease
C. Xanthinuria
D. Chloramphenicol intoxication
E. Talc and cornstarch emboli and drug abuse

Ref. JAMA
219:49, January 3, 1972

DEAFNESS AND THE AMINOGLYCOSIDES

583. OTOTOXICITY IS A WELL ESTABLISHED COMPLICATION OF THE USE OF THE AMINOGLYCOSIDE ANTIBIOTICS (STREPTOMYCIN, KANAMYCIN AND NEOMYCIN). EACH OF THE FOLLOWING IS TRUE, EXCEPT:
A. Renal failure increases the hazard of ototoxicity from the aminoglycosides
B. Ototoxicity has not been reported following the oral or colonic use of the aminoglycosides
C. Recent evidence suggests a combined ototoxic effect from the simultaneous use of ethacrynic acid and the aminoglycoside antibiotics in uremia
D. Permanent deafness has followed the use of ethacrynic acid in azotemic patients
E. Hearing loss from the use of the aminoglycosides has been commonly but not always preceded by vestibular symptoms

Ref. N Engl J Med
280:1223, May 29, 1969

PAPILLOMATOSIS

584. PAPILLOMATOSIS OF THE LARYNX IS A FAIRLY COMMON DISEASE OF CHILDREN. EACH OF THE FOLLOWING IS CORRECT IN REGARD TO MULTIPLE PAPILLOMATOSIS OF THE LOWER RESPIRATORY TRACT, EXCEPT:
A. Hemoptysis has not been noted in children with papillomatosis of the lower airway
B. The usual presenting symptoms of tracheal involvement are dyspnea and suffocation
C. Involvement of the lower respiratory tract without laryngeal lesions is very rare
D. When the disease starts during childhood, it usually appears to be self-limiting when properly managed
E. In adults the disease usually runs a more protracted course with a higher risk of developing cancer

Ref. Cancer
22:1173, December, 1968

PAPILLOMA, JUVENILE, OF THE LARYNX

585. JUVENILE LARYNGEAL PAPILLOMA MAY BE LIFE-THREATENING AND OFTEN REQUIRE PROLONGED HOSPITALIZATION FOR TREATMENT. IT IS THE MOST COMMON LOCAL NEOPLASM OF THE LARYNX IN CHILDREN, AND IT MAY PRODUCE SERIOUS UPPER AIRWAY OBSTRUCTION. JUVENILE LARYNGEAL PAPILLOMA HAVE BEEN ASSOCIATED WITH ALL OF THE FOLLOWING IN SMALL INFANTS, EXCEPT:

A. Recurrence
B. Spontaneous regression
C. Venereal warts in either or both parents
D. Aphonia
E. Malignant change

Ref. Am J Dis Child
121:417, May, 1971

TONSILLECTOMY

586. ONE OF THE FEW REMAINING INDICATIONS FOR A T AND A IS THE RARE CHILD WITH SEVERE CHRONIC UPPER AIRWAY OBSTRUCTION. EACH OF THE FOLLOWING STATEMENTS IS CONSISTENT WITH THIS SYNDROME, EXCEPT:

A. Congestive heart failure
B. Dilatation of the pulmonary vasculature
C. Pulmonary artery pressures which approximate systemic levels in some children
D. Hypercapnea and intermittent somnolence
E. Right ventricular hypertrophy

Ref. Clin Pediatr
10:236, April, 1971

FOR EACH OF THE FOLLOWING QUESTIONS, SELECT THE ONE APPROPRIATE ANSWER BY USING THE KEY OUTLINED BELOW:

1. If A, B and C are correct
2. If A and C are correct
3. If B and D are correct
4. If all are correct
5. If all are incorrect

EYE IN THE "BATTERED CHILD SYNDROME"

587. ALL INFANTS SUSPECTED OF BEING "BATTERED BABIES" SHOULD BE REFERRED TO AN OPHTHALMOLOGIST FOR COMPLETE OCULAR EXAMINATION. EARLY AND LATE OCULAR FINDINGS IN THIS SYNDROME HAVE INCLUDED WHICH OF THE FOLLOWING?:

A. Retinal hemorrhage
B. Optic atrophy
C. Posterior subcapsular cataracts
D. Retinal detachment
E. Macular scarring

Ref. Br Med J
3:398, August 14, 1971

INTRACRANIAL HYPERTENSION

588. A 16 YEAR-OLD GIRL WITH ACNE IS SEEN BECAUSE OF A FIVE DAY HISTORY OF HEADACHE, DIZZINESS, NAUSEA AND OCCASIONAL VOMITING. BILATERAL PAPILLEDEMA WITH SUPERFICIAL HEMORRHAGES IS PRESENT. ALL FINDINGS SUBSIDED WHEN WHICH OF THE FOLLOWING DRUGS WERE INTERRUPTED?:

A. Vitamin A
B. Amphetamines
C. Tetracycline
D. Marihuana
E. Barbiturates

Ref. Am J Ophthalmol
72:981, November, 1971

RETINOPATHY AND CONGENITAL HEART DISEASE

589. THE MAJORITY OF CHILDREN WITH CYANOTIC CONGENITAL HEART DISEASE DEMONSTRATE WHICH OF THE FOLLOWING ABNORMALITIES ON OPHTHALMOLOGIC EXAMINATION?:

A. Retinal hemorrhages
B. Dilated and tortuous veins
C. Dilated arterioles
D. Papilledema
E. Vasoconstriction

Ref. Pediatrics
49:243, 1972

RETINOPATHY AND CONGENITAL HEART DISEASE - Part 2

590. THE RETINOPATHY OF CYANOTIC HEART DISEASE APPEARS TO BE RELATED TO WHICH OF THE FOLLOWING?:

A. Decreased arterial oxygen saturation
B. Hypercapnia
C. Increased hematocrit
D. Increased venous pressure
E. Increased intracranial pressure

Ref. Pediatrics
49:243, 1972

OTITIS MEDIA AND TUBERCULOSIS

591. WHICH OF THE FOLLOWING SERVE AS CLINICAL CLUES IN TUBERCULOUS OTITIS MEDIA?:

A. Most children are under one year of age
B. Lack of pain
C. Profound hearing loss
D. Facial palsy
E. Postauricular fistula

Ref. J Pediatr
79:1004, December, 1971
Arch Otolaryngol
95:109, February, 1972

EYE SYNDROMES

MATCH THE SYNDROMES AND SYSTEMIC DISEASES WITH THE MOST APPROPRIATE EYE FINDINGS:

A. Tetracycline intoxication
B. Galactosemia
C. Homocystinuria
D. Wilson's disease
E. Familial dysautonomia
F. Neurofibromatosis
G. Sturge-Weber's disease
H. Chloramphenicol intoxication

592. ___ Brown-green ring at the periphery of the cornea
593. ___ Optic neuritis
594. ___ "Oil droplet" appearance of lens nucleus
595. ___ Ectopia lentis
596. ___ Papilledema
597. ___ Congenital glaucoma
598. ___ Iris nodules
599. ___ Sleeping with eyes open

Ref. DM
February, 1971

FOR EACH OF THE FOLLOWING MULTIPLE CHOICE QUESTIONS, SELECT THE ONE APPROPRIATE ANSWER:

ACHONDROPLASIA AND HYDROCEPHALUS

600. THE ETIOLOGY OF HYDROCEPHALUS IN ACHONDROPLASIA HAS BEEN STUDIED BY CISTERNOGRAPHY AND HAS BEEN ATTRIBUTED TO WHICH OF THE FOLLOWING?:

A. Localized obliteration of the subarachnoid space
B. Maldevelopment of the cranial base (chondocranium)
C. Mechanical block in the area of the tentorial hiatus
D. Constriction of the subarachnoid space in the area of the foramen magnum
E. No cause has been established

Ref. Pediatrics
49:46, January, 1972

ANOMALIES, SPINAL

601. AGENESIS OF THE LOWER SPINE (ABSENCE OF THE LUMBO-SACRAL AND COCCYGEAL VETEBRAL BODIES) SHOULD SUGGEST:

A. Congenital rubella
B. Maternal diabetes
C. Trisomy 13
D. Irradiation during pregnancy
E. Aminopterin-induced syndrome

Ref. Pediatrics
35:989, June, 1965

ARTHRALGIA AND ANEMIA

602. THE LEAST LIKELY DIAGNOSIS IN A 3 YEAR-OLD CHILD WITH SYMMETRIC ARTHRALGIA IN THE LARGE JOINTS AND A HEMATOCRIT OF 26 WOULD BE:

A. Acute leukemia
B. Metastatic neuroblastoma
C. Rheumatoid arthritis
D. Sickle cell disease
E. Metastic embryonal rhabdomysarcoma

Ref. N Engl J Med
286:208, January 27, 1972

ARTHRITIS AND CHRONIC ACTIVE HEPATITIS

603. CHILDREN WITH CHRONIC ACTIVE HEPATITIS (PLASMA CELL OR LUPOID HEPATITIS) MAY HAVE A VARIETY OF RHEUMATIC COMPLAINTS WHICH HAVE BEEN CHARACTERIZED BY ALL OF THE FOLLOWING, EXCEPT:

A. Absence of the Australia antigen in all children
B. Chronic and usually severe liver disease
C. Mild and generally transient joint disease
D. Increased levels of serum immunoglobulins although occasionally decreased levels of serum IgA
E. Occasionally, positive antinuclear and rheumatoid factors

Ref. J Pediatr
79:139, July, 1971

ARTHRITIS, GONOCOCCAL

604. GONOCOCCAL ARTHRITIS IS BECOMING MORE COMMON IN THE ADOLESCENT PATIENT. THE MOST IMPORTANT REASON FOR SERIOUS DELAYS IN INSTITUTING PROPER TREATMENT HAS BEEN:
A. Failure or a delay in studying joint fluid
B. Absence of fever in many patients
C. A normal leukocyte count
D. Lack of a history of recent sexual exposure
E. A history of preceding trauma

Ref. JAMA
217:204, July 12, 1971

ARTHRITIS, MENINGOCOCCAL

605. A SPECTRUM OF JOINT INVOLVEMENT IS SEEN IN CHILDREN WITH MENINGOCOCCAL INFECTIONS. ALL OF THE FOLLOWING CLINICAL OBSERVATIONS ARE CORRECT, EXCEPT:
A. Septic arthritis is an occasional manifestation of meningococcemia without meningitis
B. The patient may present with polyarthritis without effusion during the acute septicemia
C. The child may have a delayed joint effusion which appears a week after the acute meningococcal disease has subsided
D. The delayed joint effusions are seen in the larger joints and are extremely painful
E. The clinical response of the delayed variety of meningococcal arthritis is not affected by the administration of antibiotics

Ref. Arthritis Rheum
13:272, May, June, 1970

ARTHRITIS, SUPPURATIVE OF HIP JOINT IN INFANCY

606. WHICH OF THE FOLLOWING HAVE HAD FREQUENT ASSOCIATION WITH SUPPURATIVE ARTHRITIS OF THE HIP JOINT IN INFANCY?:
A. Femoral venipuncture
B. Neonatal jaundice
C. Dislocation of the hip
D. Hyperpyrexia
E. Absence of complications with antibiotics and drainage

Ref. J Bone Joint Surg
53A:538, 1971

OSTEOMYLITIS, ACUTE HEMATOGENOUS

607. IN A REVIEW OF 85 CASES OF ACUTE HEMATOGENOUS OSTEOMYELITIS IN INFANCY AND CHILDHOOD, THE MOST HELPFUL CLINICAL OR LABORATORY FINDING TO SUPPORT THE EARLY DIAGNOSIS WAS:
A. X-ray
B. Presence of leukocytosis
C. Elevated erythrocyte sedimentation rate
D. Localized tenderness and swelling
E. Presence of erythema and local heat

Ref. Clin Pediatr
10:377, July, 1971

JUVENILE RHEUMATOID ARTHRITIS

608. ASPIRIN CONTINUES TO BE THE DRUG OF CHOICE IN THE MANAGEMENT OF JUVENILE RHEUMATOID ARTHRITIS. THE THERAPY POSES MANY PROBLEMS IN THE ATTEMPT TO PREVENT CRIPPLING DEFORMITY AND DISABILITY. EACH OF THE FOLLOWING IS CORRECT, EXCEPT:

A. Immobilization in a cylindrical plaster cast is ideal therapy in monoarticular disease to prevent weight bearing and to preserve joint function during the acute phase
B. Patients who have been treated with both steroids and salicylates are at risk of acute salicylism when steroids are abruptly tapered
C. Eosinophilia may herald toxicity from gold therapy
D. Steroids are indicated only for the seriously ill child whose disease poses an imminent threat to life or vision
E. Chloroquine is especially dangerous in children and retinal toxicity and visual deterioration are serious complications

Ref. J Pediatr
77:355, September, 1970

SEPTIC ARTHRITIS

609. SEPTIC ARTHRITIS IN CHILDREN IS CHARACTERIZED BY ALL OF THE FOLLOWING, EXCEPT:

A. The hip is involved more than twice as frequently as any other joint
B. Most children with septic arthritis of the hip are less than two years of age
C. Early institution of drainage of the hip joint is urgent because of the potential for destruction of the capital femoral epiphysis and pathologic dislocation
D. Injection of antibiotics directly into the joint space is necessary to obtain adequate concentration of antibiotics such as methicillin, ampicillin, penicillin and cephalothin
E. Septic arthritis may complicate osteomyelitis through direct extension

Ref. N Engl J Med
284:349, February 18, 1971

SHOULDER PAIN IN A 12-YEAR-OLD

610. AN AFEBRILE 12 YEAR-OLD BOY DEVELOPED SUDDEN PAIN IN HIS LEFT SHOULDER 3-1/2 WEEKS PRIOR TO A ROENTGENOGRAM WHICH DEMONSTRATED WIDENING OF THE RADIOLUCENT LINE OF THE EPIPHYSEAL CARTILAGE OF THE PROXIMAL HUMERUS WITH SOME OSTEOPOROSIS OF THE PROXIMAL QUARTER INCH OF THE DIAPHYSIS ADJACENT TO THE LINE. THE MOST LIKELY DIAGNOSIS IS:

A. Acute lymphoblastic leukemia
B. Osteomyelitis
C. Metastatic neuroblastoma
D. Osteogenic sarcoma
E. Little league pitching

Ref. Pediatrics
49:267, 1972

SYNOVITIS, HIP

611. TRANSIENT SYNOVITIS OF THE HIP IS THE MOST COMMON CAUSE OF PAINFUL HIP IN CHILDREN. AFTER A REMISSION, RECURRENCE OF PAIN, LIMP, OR RESTRICTED HIP MOTION SHOULD SUGGEST THE POSSIBILITY OF:

A. Rheumatoid arthritis
B. Rheumatic fever
C. Legg-Calvé-Perthes' disease
D. Osteoid osteoma of the femoral neck
E. Slipped femoral capital epiphysis

Ref. Pediatrics 47:558, 1971

SYPHILIS, CONGENITAL

612. A THREE WEEK OLD INFANT WITH INABILITY TO MOVE HIS UPPER EXTREMITIES DEMONSTRATES ON X-RAY EXAMINATION PERIOSTITIS OF BOTH HUMERI ASSOCIATED WITH DESTRUCTIVE METAPHYSEAL LESIONS AND A PATHOLOGIC FRACTURE OF THE RIGHT HUMERAL DIAPHYSIS. THERE IS GENERALIZED LYMPHADENOPATHY AND HEPATOSPLENOMEGALY. THE HEMOGLOBIN IS 8.0 gms AND THE INFANT HAS "FAILED TO THRIVE." THE MOST IMPORTANT DIAGNOSTIC CLUE WOULD BE REVEALED IN:

A. Demonstration of anti-treponemal IgM fluorescent antibodies for congenital syphilis
B. Bone marrow examination
C. "Battered-child" workup
D. Lymph node biopsy
E. Bone biopsy

Ref. Infect Dis 1:11. June, 1971

FOR EACH OF THE FOLLOWING QUESTIONS, SELECT THE ONE APPROPRIATE ANSWER BY USING THE KEY OUTLINED BELOW:

1. If A, B and C are correct
2. If A and C are correct
3. If B and D are correct
4. If all are correct
5. If all are incorrect

DUCHENNE'S MUSCULAR DYSTROPHY

613. 15 TO 20 PER CENT OF FEMALE CARRIERS OF THE GENE FOR DUCHENNE'S MUSCULAR DYSTROPHY REMAIN UNDETECTED BY PRESENT TECHNIQUES. WHICH OF THE FOLLOWING HAVE BEEN SHOWN TO BE OF VALUE IN DETECTING 100 PER CENT OF CARRIERS OF THE GENE?:

A. Rubidium chloride Rb 86
B. Total body potassium concentration
C. Electromyography
D. Immunoelectrophoresis of serum
E. Serum creatine phosphokinase

Ref. Arch Neurol 25:193, September, 1971

OSTEOMYELITIS OF THE PATELLA

614. OSTEOMYELITIS OF THE PATELLA SHOULD BE IN THE DIFFERENTIAL DIAGNOSIS WHEN A CHILD PRESENTS WITH AN ACUTE CELLULITIS OF THE ANTERIOR KNEE. WHICH OF THE FOLLOWING ARE CORRECT IN RELATION TO THIS CLINICAL ENTITY?:
A. Suppurative arthritis of the knee joint is a common complication in children
B. The clinical course is usually septic
C. The earliest roentgenologic sign in children is periosteal elevation
D. Osteomyelitis of the patella, unlike other bones, is rarely caused by staphylococcus aureus
E. Most cases occur in children of four years or younger

Ref. Clin Pediatr
10:577, October, 1971

CARPALS, ABNORMALITIES

ABNORMALITIES OF THE CARPALS OCCUR IN A VARIETY OF CONGENITAL SYNDROMES. MATCH THE APPROPRIATE ANOMALY WITH THE MOST FREQUENT CLINICAL DIAGNOSIS:

615. ___ Decreased carpal angle
616. ___ Carpal fusion
617. ___ Absent or hypoplastic capitate
618. ___ Scaphoid fused to other carpals
619. ___ Absent or hypoplastic scaphoid
620. ___ Extra distal carpals

A. Diastrophic dwarfism
B. Dyschondrosteosis
C. Ellis-Van Crevald
D. Epiphyseal dysplasia
E. Fanconi's anemia
F. Holt-Oram

Ref. Am J Roentgenol Radium Ther Nucl Med
CXII:443, July, 1971

THUMBS, ABNORMALITIES

ANOMALIES OF THE THUMB AND THE PATTERN OF THUMB DEVELOPMENT MAY BE HELPFUL IN ARRIVING AT A DIAGNOSIS. MATCH THE FOLLOWING THUMB ABNORMALITIES WITH THEIR MOST FREQUENT SYNDROME ASSOCIATION:

621. ___ Macrodactyly
622. ___ Triphalangeal
623. ___ Short and proximally placed
624. ___ Broad
625. ___ Hypoplasia and aplasia

A. Holt-Oram
B. Neurofibromatosis
C. Rubinstein-Taybi
D. Cornelia de Lange

Ref. Radiology
100:115, July, 1971

FOR EACH OF THE FOLLOWING MULTIPLE CHOICE QUESTIONS, SELECT THE ONE APPROPRIATE ANSWER:

AMNION NODOSUM

626. AMNION NODOSUM REPRESENTS A "GRANULOMATOUS" NODULE WHICH CONTAINS DESQUAMATED EPIDERMAL CELLS AND HAIRS. IT APPEARS TO REPRESENT A REACTION TO VERNIX WHICH HAS DROPPED TO THE SURFACE OF THE PLACENTA AND IS PATHOGNOMONIC FOR OLIGOHYDRAMNIOS. IT HAS BEEN ASSOCIATED WITH ALL OF THE FOLLOWING, EXCEPT:
A. Death and retention of the fetus
B. Severe obstructive uropathy
C. Renal agenesis
D. Prolonged rupture of the fetal membranes
E. Postmaturity

Ref. Path of Human Placenta
Page 44, 1967
Blanc, W.A.

BLOOD GASES

627. AN ARTERIAL BLOOD SAMPLE FROM THE UMBILICUS IN A ONE DAY-OLD INFANT REVEALS A pH OF 7.35, PCO_2 OF 58 mm Hg, AND A HCO_3 OF 28.0 mEq/L. THIS WOULD SUGGEST WHICH OF THE FOLLOWING ACID-BASE STATES?:
A. Mixed metabolic and respiratory acidosis
B. Partially compensated metabolic acidosis
C. Uncompensated metabolic acidosis
D. Compensated respiratory acidosis
E. Uncompensated respiratory acidosis

Ref. Pediatr Clin N Am
17:902, November, 1970

CYANOSIS IN NEWBORN

628. 100 PER CENT OXYGEN BREATHING IN A CYANOTIC NEWBORN INFANT CANNOT IMPROVE:
A. A large intracardiac or intrapulmonary right-to-left shunt
B. Alveolar hypoventilation
C. Severe ventilation/perfusion unevenness
D. An infant with a large patent ductus arteriosus
E. An infant with increased pulmonary blood flow

Ref. J Pediatr
77:488, September, 1970

CYANOSIS IN NEWBORN

629. AN AGGRESSIVE DIAGNOSTIC APPROACH TO AN INFANT WITH CYANOSIS IS IMPORTANT SINCE TREATMENT IS AVAILABLE IN THE MAJORITY OF INSTANCES. ALL OF THE FOLLOWING IS CORRECT IN REGARD TO THE RESPIRATORY PATTERN OF NEWBORN INFANTS, EXCEPT:
A. A marked increase in respiratory rate in a cyanotic baby suggests a pulmonary cause, left-sided heart failure, or pulmonary overcirculation
B. Cyanosis with increased depth of respiration suggests congenital heart disease with underperfused lungs
C. Intercostal retractions suggest airway obstruction
D. Cyanosis with marked periodic breathing or apneic spells suggests central nervous system disease with alveolar hypoventilation
E. Flaring of the alae nasi and grunting are pathognomonic in a newborn for right-to-left shunting and increased pulmonary blood flow

Ref. J Pediatr
77:487, September, 1970

630. IMMERSION OF A BABY'S HEEL IN A WATER AT 100° F. PRODUCES VASODILATION AND WILL HELP DISTINGUISH CENTRAL FROM PERIPHERAL CYANOSIS. EACH OF THE FOLLOWING IS CORRECT IN REGARD TO THE EXAMINATION OF BLOOD OBTAINED FROM A DEEP HEEL PRICK OF A WELL-WARMED FOOT, EXCEPT:
A. If the color of the blood is bright red the possibility of central cyanosis is eliminated
B. A Dextrostix test provides a screening test for hypoglycemia as a contributing factor to central cyanosis
C. Methemoglobinemia may be suspected by failure of blood to become red when placed on a slide and exposed to room air
D. Measurement of capillary PAO_2 is accurate since the oxygen tension of the blood is unaffected by exposure to room air
E. If the blood is free flowing and can be collected anaerobically from the center of drops of blood, one may obtain a rough indication of oxygen tension

Ref. J Pediatr
77:488, September, 1970

EARLY DISCHARGE OF HIGH RISK NEONATES

631. THE SAFETY OF EARLY DISCHARGE OF A HIGH-RISK INFANT OR ONE WHO IS "SMALL-FOR-DATES" APPEARS TO DEPEND LEAST ON:
A. Vital signs which are stable in a normal room environment
B. Early maternal contact and participation in the care of the infant
C. Vigorous appetite on breast or formula
D. Absence of disease
E. Attainment of a weight of five pounds

Ref. Clin Pediatr
10:467, August, 1971

FETAL LUNG FLUID, DISAPPEARANCE OF

632. FETAL LUNG CONTAINS WATER IN THE EXTRAVASCULAR SPACES PRIOR TO THE ONSET OF EXTRA-UTERINE RESPIRATIONS. FOLLOWING BIRTH, ALL THE FLUID IN THE POTENTIAL AIR SPACES MUST BE REMOVED BEFORE GAS EXCHANGE CAN OCCUR. EACH OF THE FOLLOWING IS CORRECT, EXCEPT:

A. Extravascular fluid in the lungs of newborn rabbits disappears slowly over a period of days rather than hours
B. The rate of disappearance of extravascular fluid from the lungs was the same in rabbits delivered by vagina or by cesarean section
C. Lung blood volume did not change following birth
D. Extravascular fluid disappears from the lungs via the pulmonary capillaries
E. Extravascular fluid disappears from the lungs via the lymphatics

Ref. J Pediatr
78:837, May, 1971

HYALINE MEMBRANE DISEASE

633. THE DIAGNOSIS OF HYALINE MEMBRANE DISEASE IS RARELY DIFFICULT BUT ITS BASIC CAUSE HAS NOT BEEN DEFINED. EACH OF THE FOLLOWING IS CORRECT, EXCEPT:

A. Perinatal asphyxia is a prerequisite to the development of hyaline membrane disease
B. There is a familial tendency in the development of hyaline membrane disease
C. Hyaline membrane disease is not related to delivery by cesarean section per se, but to the indications for cesarean section
D. Racial factors have not been accurately identified in hyaline membrane disease
E. Maternal diabetes is not necessarily a predisposing factor, except as it leads to premature delivery

Ref. Pediatr Clin N Am
17:943, November, 1970

634. IN HYALINE MEMBRANE DISEASE ALL OF THE FOLLOWING ARE CORRECT, EXCEPT:

A. Right-to-left shunting of blood occurs across the foramen ovale and the ductus arteriosus
B. Heart failure is commonly seen in hyaline membrane disease
C. The claim that delayed cord-clamping has improved the mortality and morbidity has been largely discounted
D. Peripheral and pulmonary hypotension is the hallmark of hyaline membrane disease
E. The lungs show widespread atelectasis

Ref. Pediatr Clin N Am
17:946, November, 1970

ADRENAL AND HYALINE MEMBRANE DISEASE

635. PERINATAL MORTALITY RATES CONTINUE TO BE STRONGLY INFLUENCED BY HYALINE MEMBRANE DISEASE. ADEQUATE ANIMAL MODELS EXIST (THE PREMATURELY DELIVERED LAMB OR PRIMATE) FOR THE STUDY OF THIS PROBLEM. ALL OF THE FOLLOWING ARE CORRECT, EXCEPT:
A. Evidence in the anencephalic newborn suggests that cortisol transfer from the mother does not take place since 17-OH corticosteroid levels are far below normal
B. Pulmonary surfactant activity is decreased in the lungs and lung fluid of infants with hyaline membrane disease
C. There is indirect evidence that the adult zone of the adrenal cortex has a role in surfactant production through its elaboration of corticosteroids
D. There appears to be a correlation between the relative size of the adrenal glands and the presence of hyaline membrane disease in newborn infants
E. There is need for caution in the use of corticosteroids as prophylaxis against hyaline membrane disease in high risk gestations

Ref. Pediatrics 47:650, April, 1971

HYALINE MEMBRANE DISEASE

636. ADAPTATION FROM INTRA-UTERINE TO EXTRA-UTERINE LIFE IS A DRAMATIC AND COMPLEX EVENT WHICH IS OFTEN COMPLICATED BY A WIDE VARIETY OF RESPIRATORY PROBLEMS. EACH OF THE FOLLOWING IS CORRECT IN RESPECT TO HYALINE MEMBRANE DISEASE (HMD), EXCEPT:
A. Almost all infants who have hyaline membrane disease are born before 38 weeks gestation
B. Most infants with HMD require resuscitation at birth
C. Abnormal respirations are rarely present in the first hour of life
D. The maternal history is often complicated by antepartum uterine bleeding, anemia or delivery by cesarean section before the onset of labor
E. Apgar scores are usually below 7 at one and five minutes

Ref. Pediatrics 47:758, April, 1971

637. AMONG LIVE BORN INFANTS, THE SINGLE MOST IMPORTANT CAUSE OF MORTALITY IN THE FIRST WEEK OF LIFE IS:
A. Sepsis and meningitis
B. Hyaline membrane disease
C. Congenital abnormalities
D. Hemolytic disease of the newborn
E. Intra-uterine anoxia

Ref. Pediatr Clin N Am 17:943, November, 1970

HYPOTHERMIA OF NEWBORN

638. HYPOTHERMIA AND COLD INJURY OF THE NEWBORN HAS BEEN ASSOCIATED WITH ALL OF THE FOLLOWING CLINICAL OBSERVATIONS, EXCEPT:
A. Hypoglycemia
B. Metabolic acidosis
C. Edema
D. Complete A-V dissociation by electrocardiography
E. Optimum responses to treatment when hypothermia is rapidly corrected

Ref. N Engl J Med 285:332, August 5, 1971

NARCOTIC ADDICTION, NEONATAL

639. IN A STUDY OF 384 INFANTS BORN TO 382 HEROIN ADDICTED MOTHERS ALL OF THE FOLLOWING WERE OBSERVED, EXCEPT:
A. Increase in congenital abnormalities
B. Decreased incidence of hyperbilirubinemia compared to a general newborn population
C. Increased incidence of low birth weight infants
D. A correlation between the length of maternal addiction and the incidence of withdrawal signs in the infant
E. Control of all of the withdrawal signs in the newborn infant with chlorpromazine

Ref. Pediatrics 48:188, August, 1971

640. IN NEONATAL NARCOTIC ADDICTION ALL OF THE FOLLOWING SIGNS OF WITHDRAWAL ARE OBSERVED, EXCEPT:
A. Irritability
B. Edema
C. Tremors
D. Vomiting
E. Sneezing

Ref. Pediatrics 48:185, August, 1971

HYPONATREMIA

641. HYPONATREMIA IN THE NEWBORN IS MOST LIKELY TO BE ASSOCIATED WITH:
A. Relative or absolute water overloading
B. Increased renal tubular loss of sodium after relief of obstructive uropathy
C. Deficiency of adrenal mineralocorticoids
D. Administration of diuretics to the mother during pregnancy
E. Inappropriate antidiuretic hormone secretion in the infant

Ref. N Engl J Med 284:660, March 25, 1971

JAUNDICE AND FLANK MASSES

642. A 14 DAY-OLD INFANT WITH BILATERAL FLANK MASSES AND PROLONGED NEONATAL JAUNDICE WAS NOTED BY INTRAVENOUS PYELOGRAM TO HAVE SUPRARENAL, AVASCULAR AND SHARPLY DEFINED MASSES WHICH WERE SURROUNDED BY A FAINT RIM OF CALCIFICATION. THE DIAGNOSIS IN THIS AND TWO OTHER INFANTS HAS BEEN PROVEN TO BE ASSOCIATED WITH:
A. Bilateral massive adrenal hemorrhage
B. Neonatal neuroblastoma
C. Wolman's xanthomatosis
D. Renal duplications with upper pole hydronephrosis
E. Congenital adrenal hyperplasia

Ref. Radiology 98:263, 1971

PHYSIOLOGIC JAUNDICE

643. EXPERIMENTAL WORK WITH NEWBORN MONKEYS HAS LENT SUPPORT TO THE THEORY THAT THE MOST LIKELY EXPLANATION OF PHYSIOLOGIC JAUNDICE OF THE NEWBORN IS:
A. Increased bilirubin production (as with a shortened life span of the erythrocyte)
B. Deficient hepatic uptake (cell membrane defect or cytoplasmic protein defect)
C. Deficient hepatic conjugation of bilirubin to bilirubin glucuronide
D. Deficient hepatic excretion of bilirubin
E. Increased reabsorption of bilirubin via the enterohepatic circulation
Ref. N Engl J Med
283:1, January 7, 1971

PREGNANCY, HIGH-RISK

644. PREDICTABLE PREMATURE BIRTHS ARE MOST COMMON IN WOMEN WITH A HISTORY OF:
A. One or more spontaneous abortions
B. Previous delivery of a low-birthweight infant
C. One or more perinatal deaths
D. More than four pregnancies
E. No previous premature births
Ref. Hospital Practice
6:133, October, 1971

OXYGEN IN PREMATURES

645. PEDIATRICIANS USE OXYGEN CONCENTRATIONS ABOVE 40 PER CENT IN INFANTS WITH RESPIRATORY DISTRESS BECAUSE OF THE GENERAL IMPRESSION THAT RETROLENTAL FIBROPLASIA WILL NOT OCCUR IF THE ARTERIAL pO_2 IS KEPT WITHIN "SAFE" LIMITS. EACH OF THE FOLLOWING IS CORRECT, EXCEPT:
A. Cyanosis usually appears when the oxygen saturation of hemoglobin falls below 80 per cent
B. Above 90 per cent oxygen saturation, large increases in pO_2 produce only small increments in percentage saturation
C. Values below 40 mm Hg with an infant breathing 100 per cent oxygen require the use of a respirator for infants of less than 1500 grams
D. Clinical estimates of pO_2 levels are predictable in pink infants
E. Sudden rises in arterial pO_2 levels with the same ambient oxygen concentration may occur in infants in centrally mediated respiratory distress
Ref. Pediatr Clin N Am
17:, May, 1970

OXYGEN THERAPY FOR NEWBORNS

646. CURRENT RECOMMEMDATIONS FOR THE ADMINISTRATION OF OXYGEN TO NEWBORN INFANTS HAVE SUGGESTED ALL OF THE FOLLOWING, EXCEPT:

A. Oxygen tension of arterial blood should not exceed 100 mm mercury and should be maintained between 60 and 80 mm mercury
B. If blood gas measurements are not available, a mature infant who is not apneic but has generalized cyanosis may be given oxygen in a concentration just high enough to abolish the cyanosis
C. The regulation of inspired oxygen concentration to an immature infant should be based on blood gas measurements
D. It is unnecessary to warm, and humidify mixtures of oxygen and room air when delivered to an infant by endotracheal tube or mask
E. The ideal sites for arterial oxygen tension studies are the radial or temporal arteries

Ref. Standards and Recommendations for Hospital Care of Newborn Infants, Am Acad Pediatr, 1971

PHOTOTHERAPY IN ABO INCOMPATIBILITY

647. IN THE USE OF PHOTOTHERAPY IN ABO INCOMPATIBILITY ALL OF THE FOLLOWING HAVE BEEN OBSERVED, EXCEPT:

A. The photodecomposition of bilirubin is greatest in the blue spectral region between 420 and 490 nm
B. Phototherapy is as effective in infants of low birth weight as in those of greater weight and maturity
C. Phototherapy is not as useful and as effective in Negro infants as in Caucasians
D. Phototherapy reduces the need for exchange transfusion in the treatment of ABO incompatibility
E. The appearance of the skin is not a reliable index of the response to phototherapy

Ref. J Pediatr 79:904, December, 1971

PNEUMOTHORAX IN NEWBORN INFANTS

648. IN THE NEWBORN INFANT PNEUMOTHORAX IS MOST COMMONLY ASSOCIATED WITH:

A. Hyaline membrane disease
B. Pneumonia
C. Meconium aspiration syndrome
D. Resuscitation
E. Caesarean section

Ref. J Pediatr 80:98, January, 1972

649. ALTHOUGH ROENTGENOGRAMS ARE ESSENTIAL IN THE DIAGNOSIS OF PNEUMOTHORAX IN THE NEWBORN INFANT, WHICH OF THE FOLLOWING MAY BE THE MOST USEFUL TECHNIQUE OR OBSERVATION IN THE EARLY DETECTION OF THIS COMPLICATION IN HIGH-RISK BABIES?:

A. Electrocardiographic oscilloscope monitoring
B. Repeated auscultation of the chest
C. Apnea monitoring
D. Development of grunting respirations
E. Onset of cyanosis

Ref. J Pediatr 80:98, January, 1972

R FACTORS AND THE NEWBORN

650. IT HAS BEEN SUGGESTED THAT AT LEAST 50 PER CENT OF ENTEROBACTERIAL ISOLATES ARE RESISTANT TO MULTIPLE ANTIBIOTICS AS A RESULT OF R FACTORS. ALL OF THE FOLLOWING ARE CORRECT, EXCEPT:

A. R factors are extrachromosomal genetic materials that may be transferred from an organism of the same or different species by cell to cell contact
B. The recipient cell is capable of donating the acquired R factor
C. E.coli isolated from babies in a "high-risk" nursery have a high degree of antibiotic resistance
D. Infants in a "high-risk" unit show a high colonization rate of the upper respiratory tract with gram-negative antibiotic-resistant bacteria
E. Antibiotic-resistant enteric organisms with R factors are rarely recovered from the feces of neonates who are less than five days of age

Ref. J Pediatr 80:198, February, 1972

SEPSIS, NEONATAL

651. A TECHNIQUE WHICH CAN MOST QUICKLY SUPPORT THE PEDIATRICIAN'S SUSPICION OF INTRA-UTERINE BACTERIAL SEPSIS:

A. Demonstration of three or more polymorphonuclear leukocytes per high-power field in smear of infant's external ear canal
B. Culture of infant's external ear canal
C. Urine culture obtained by suprapubic tap
D. Culture of gastric contents
E. Blood culture

Ref. J Pediatr 79:247, August, 1971

SMALL FOR DATES, GROWTH HORMONE

652. IN STUDIES OF FULL-TERM INFANTS WHO ARE SMALL FOR GESTATIONAL AGE, ALL OF THE FOLLOWING OBSERVATIONS HAVE BEEN MADE, EXCEPT:

A. Growth hormone deficiency does not appear to be related to neonatal hypoglycemia
B. Growth hormone levels appear to rise in the first days of life in response to the first postnatal feedings
C. Growth hormone deficiency does not appear to contribute to the small size of the infant
D. In a 2-year study of the growth patterns of full-term infants who were small for gestational age the data is highly suggestive that the growth hormone in these children is biologically inactive
E. The length and head growth of the full-term infant who is small for dates are usually less affected than birth weight

Ref. Pediatrics 48:190, August, 1971

FOR EACH OF THE FOLLOWING QUESTIONS, SELECT THE ONE APPROPRIATE ANSWER BY USING THE KEY OUTLINED BELOW:

1. If A, B and C are correct
2. If A and C are correct
3. If B and D are correct
4. If all are correct
5. If all are incorrect

ABO ERYTHROBLASTOSIS

653. WHICH OF THE FOLLOWING CRITERIA SHOULD BE FOLLOWED IN ESTABLISHING A DIAGNOSIS OF ABO INCOMPATIBILITY IN THE NEWBORN?:
A. Fetal-maternal ABO incompatibility
B. Microspherocytosis
C. Reduced red cell acetylcholinesterase activity
D. Negative antiglobulin test (direct or indirect)
E. Clinical icterus in the first 48 hours of life
Ref. J Pediatr
79:912, December, 1971

ABORTIONS, SPONTANEOUS

654. IN A REPORT BY THE WORLD HEALTH ORGANIZATION ON SPONTANEOUS ABORTION, WHICH OF THE FOLLOWING OBSERVATIONS WERE MADE?:
A. The incidence of spontaneous abortion is probably in the order of 15-20 per cent of all pregnancies
B. Almost half of all fetal deaths occur prior to the ninth week of gestation
C. 30-40 per cent of embryos recovered from spontaneous abortions are malformed
D. Most XO conceptuses are aborted spontaneously
E. The principle abnormalities identified are trisomies of autosomes, XO, and polyploidies
Ref. WHO Tech Report Series, 461, 1970

BARBITURATE WITHDRAWAL SYMPTOMS IN THE NEWBORN

655. THE SPECTRUM OF WITHDRAWAL SYMPTOMS FROM BARBITURATES IN THE NEWBORN INFANT DIFFERS FROM THOSE INDUCED BY OPIATES IN WHICH OF THE FOLLOWING RESPECTS?:
A. Good one minute Apgar scores
B. Onset of symptoms at a later age
C. Lower incidence of jaundice
D. Presence of sneezing, hiccups, yawning and mouth movements
E. Tremors
Ref. J Pediatr
80:190, February, 1972

CHROMOSOMES AND INTRA-UTERINE GROWTH FAILURE

656. INTRA-UTERINE GROWTH FAILURE IS HIGHLY CHARACTERISTIC OF RECOGNIZED CHROMOSOME ABNORMALITIES WITH THE EXCEPTION OF WHICH OF THE FOLLOWING?:
A. Poly-X syndromes
B. Trisomy 18
C. Klinefelter's
D. Gonadal dysgenesis
E. Down's
Ref. Pediatr Clin N Am
17:101, February, 1970

NEWBORN, EXPIRATORY GRUNTING

657. EXPIRATORY GRUNTING IS THE NEWBORN IS ASSOCIATED WITH WHICH OF THE FOLLOWING CLINICAL CONDITIONS?:
A. Transient tachypnea of the newborn
B. Left heart failure
C. Respiratory distress syndrome
D. Normal newborns with late clamping of the cord
E. Pneumonia

Ref. Pediatrics
48:865, December, 1971

FETAL GROWTH IMPAIRMENT

658. FOUR DISTINCT PATTERNS OF FETAL GROWTH IMPAIRMENT MAY BE IDENTIFIED BY WHICH OF THE FOLLOWING MEASUREMENTS OF NEWBORN INFANTS?:
A. Crown-heel length
B. Head circumference
C. Birth weight
D. Pelvic breadth
E. A-P roentgenograms of leg

Ref. Pediatrics
48:511, October, 1971

FETAL MEMBRANES

659. WITH RETENTION OF A DEAD FETUS IN UTERO, WHICH OF THE FOLLOWING ASSOCIATIONS HAVE BEEN OBSERVED?:
A. Loss of strength and elasticity of fetal membranes
B. An increase in the permeability of the membranes of the dead fetus to the hemoglobin molecule
C. An increase in friability of the fetal membranes
D. A gradual decline in maternal blood fibrinogen levels
E. An increased incidence of amniotic fluid embolism

Ref. Br Med J
1:492, February 27, 1971

HIGH-RISK INFANTS, TRANSFER

660. IN THE TRANSFER OF A LOW BIRTH WEIGHT OR OTHER HIGH-RISK NEWBORN INFANT TO A REFERRAL HOSPITAL, WHICH OF THE FOLLOWING PRINCIPLES SHOULD BE ADHERED TO:
A. Pneumothorax, pneumomediastinum or trapped gas in the abdomen may make it hazardous to fly, even at 5000 feet
B. A stomach tube should be used to empty the stomach before beginning the journey
C. A slow ambulance trip is preferable
D. In infant should receive one dose of 1 mg of vitamin K_1 before he is transferred
E. A specimen of the mother's blood for cross-matching should accompany the infant

Ref. Am Acad Pediatr
Page 95, 1971

INTRA-UTERINE GROWTH FAILURE

661. INTRA-UTERINE GROWTH FAILURE OR FETAL MALNUTRITION HAS BEEN ASSOCIATED WITH WHICH OF THE FOLLOWING FACTORS?:

A. Multiple births
B. Maternal cigarette smoking
C. Chromosomal anomalies
D. Viral embryopathies
E. Low socio-economics

Ref. Pediatr Clin N AM
17:9, February, 1970

NEWBORN, HOSPITAL CARE

662. IN RECOMMEMDATIONS FOR THE HOSPITAL CARE OF NEWBORN INFANTS THE AMERICAN ACADEMY OF PEDIATRICS HAS SUGGESTED WHICH OF THE FOLLOWING?:

A. Masks are not recommemded for routine use by nurses and physicians in the newborn nursery
B. There are no valid medical indications for circumcision in the neonatal period
C. Most infectious agents responsible for colonizing and infecting infants in the newborn nursery are transmitted from infant to infant by the hands of nursery personnel
D. Iodophors (water soluble complexes of iodine with surfactive agents) are superior to hexachlorophene preparations for hand washing in the nursery
E. Breast-feeding should be started as soon after delivery as the condition of the mother and infant permit

Ref. Standards and Recommendations for Hospital Care of Newborn Infants
Am Acad Pediatr 1971

PHOTOTHERAPY IN ABO INCOMPATIBILITY

663. IN THE CONTROL OF HYPERBILIRUNEMIA WHICH ACCOMPANIES ABO INCOMPATIBILITY, WHICH OF THE FOLLOWING HAVE BEEN NOTED?:

A. In light-treated infants, peak bilirubin concentrations do not occur after the third day of life
B. Phototherapy is not indicated for infants with ABO disease of mild onset and severity
C. Shielding of the infants's eyes is required
D. Infants with hemolytic disease who are treated with phototherapy should be monitored for the development of anemia
E. Phototherapy lamps lose energy in the blue spectrum after several hours of use

Ref. J Pediatr
79:904, December, 1971

THALASSEMIA AND HEMOLYTIC DISEASE OF THE NEWBORN

664. WHICH OF THE FOLLOWING ARE CORRECT IN REGARD TO HEMOLYTIC DISEASE OF THE NEWBORN AND THALASSEMIA?:
A. Hemolytic disease of the newborn is most often associated with the homozygous alpha variety of thalassemia
B. Hydrops fetalis and intra-uterine death may complicate severe hemolytic disease and thalassemia
C. Hemolysis due to homozygous beta-thalassemia does not manifest at birth
D. Gamma-beta thalassemia has been described as a cause of erythroblastosis
E. Gamma-beta thalassemia should be considered in the differential of hypochromic anemia in the newborn

Ref. N Engl J Med
286:129, January 20, 1972

TWINS, IDENTICAL OR FRATERNAL

TWINS OF THE OPPOSITE SEX ARE OBVIOUSLY FRATERNAL. HOW DO THE FOLLOWING HELP TO DISTINGUISH THE IDENTICAL OR FRATERNAL TWIN BIRTH?:

A. Identical
B. Fraternal
C. Both
D. Neither

665. ___ Two chorionic sacs
666. ___ No complete or partial dividing membrane between the fetuses
667. ___ Twin fused placentas
668. ___ Translucent septum with no chorionic tissue between the amnions
669. ___ Demonstration by microscopic examination in the "T" section of the placenta of four layers (where membranes leave the placenta to form a septum between the two fetal cavities)

Ref. Obstet Gynecol
37:538, April, 1971

FOR EACH OF THE FOLLOWING MULTIPLE CHOICE QUESTIONS, SELECT THE ONE APPROPRIATE ANSWER:

ALPHA-1-ANTITRYPSIN DEFICIENCY

670. TWO DISPARATE DISEASE STATES, AN ADULT FORM OF EMPHYSEMA AND A CHILDHOOD FORM OF LIVER CIRRHOSIS, HAVE BEEN ASSOCIATED WITH AN INHERITED ABSENCE OF ALPHA-1-ANTITRYPSIN. ALL OF THE FOLLOWING ARE CORRECT, EXCEPT:
A. Symptomatic pulmonary emphysema in childhood associated with hereditary alpha-1-antitrypsin deficiency has not been described
B. Progressive dyspnea with lack of clinical chronic bronchitis in the early stages is characteristic of the pulmonary disease
C. Several children with the deficiency state but with no pulmonary disease have been observed
D. Children with severe infantile cirrhosis and alpha-1-antitrypsin deficiency have not shown pulmonary disease
E. One of the clinical features of this type of familial emphysema has been the higher incidence in females

Ref. J Pediatr
79:20, July, 1971

EPIGLOTTITIS, ACUTE

671. THE SAFEST AND MOST RELIABLE WAY TO DIFFERENTIATE ACUTE EPIGLOTTITIS FROM THE SUBLOTTIC CROUP SYNDROME IS:
A. Direct inspection of the fiery red, swollen epiglottis at the bedside
B. Lateral neck radiographs
C. Presence of hoarseness
D. Drooling
E. Dysphagia and hyperextension of the neck

Ref. J Pediatr
80:96, January, 1972

HEMOPTYSIS

672. A 10 YEAR-OLD BOY WITH PERENNIAL ALLERGIC RHINITIS HAS A 3 YEAR HISTORY OF INTERMITTENT WHEEZING, CHRONIC COUGH RECURRENT PNEUMONIA AND HEMOPTYSIS. BRONCHOSCOPIC AND BRONCHOGRAPHIC STUDIES ARE NEGATIVE. A RIGHT BRONCHIAL ARTERIOGRAM REVEALED ENLARGED BRONCHIAL ARTERIES ACCOMPANIED BY HYPERVASCULARITY IN THE POSTERIOR BASILAR SEGMENT OF THE RIGHT LOWER LOBE. THE MOST LIKELY DIAGNOSIS IS:
A. A radiolucent foreign body
B. Bronchiectasis
C. Bronchial asthma
D. Pulmonary arteriovenous fistula
E. Cystic fibrosis

Ref. Clin Pediatr
10:479, August, 1971

PENTAMIDINE AND PNEUMOCYSTIS

673. INFECTIONS DUE TO MORE OPPORTUNISTIC AND EXOTIC ORGANISMS HAVE INCREASED IN CHILDREN WITH MALIGNANCIES WHO ARE BEING TREATED WITH RADIATION AND CHEMOTHERAPY. EACH OF THE FOLLOWING IS CORRECT REGARDING PNEUMOCYSTIS CARINII AND PENTAMIDINE, EXCEPT:

A. Pneumocystis carinii has not been cultivated in vitro
B. Pentamidine has been efficacious in the treatment of pneumocystis carinii pneumonia
C. Hypoglycemia is a complication of pentamidine therapy
D. Nephrotoxic antibiotics may be safely combined with pentamidine
E. Hemoptysis and pneumothorax have complicated pulmonary needle aspiration in the diagnosis of pneumocystis infections

Ref. JAMA
214:1067, November 9, 1970

PNEUMOCYSTIS

674. PNEUMOCYSTIS CARINII IS MOST FREQUENTLY RESPONSIBLE FOR DIFFUSE INTERSTITIAL PNEUMONIA IN CHILDREN RECEIVING IMMUNOSUPPRESSIVE DRUGS OR WITH IMMUNE DEFICIENCY DISEASES. EACH OF THE FOLLOWING STATEMENTS IS CORRECT, EXCEPT:

A. It is sometimes impossible to differentiate by radiographs the lungs of children with pneumocystis from those of cytomegalic inclusion virus
B. Fever may be absent in pneumocystis infections in children
C. Bloody sputum and pleuritic pain are rare
D. Lung biopsy is the most reliable method of diagnosing pneumocystis pneumonia
E. Pneumocysitis carinii pneumonia has been rarely diagnosed in infants

Ref. N Engl J Med
280:287, February 6, 1969

PNEUMONIA, STAPHYLOCOCCAL

675. IN A 2 TO 4 YEAR FOLLOW-UP OF CHILDREN WHO HAD HAD STAPHYLOCOCCAL PNEUMONIA IN INFANCY, WHICH OF THE FOLLOWING WAS MOST COMMONLY FOUND?:

A. Bronchiectasis
B. Restrictive lung disease
C. Pleural thickening and other residual roentgenographic abnormalities
D. Retardation of growth
E. No abnormalities of growth, pulmonary function or in roentgenograms

Ref. Amer J Dis Child
122:386, November, 1971

TUBERCULOSIS, INTERMEDIATE PPD

676. IN SKIN-TESTING ONE HUNDRED AND FIFTEEN CONSECUTIVE PATIENTS WITH ACTIVE TUBERCULOSIS WITH INTERMEDIATE STRENGTH COMMERCIAL PPD ANTIGEN, THE MOST COMMON CAUSE FOR A NEGATIVE SKIN REACTION WAS:

A. Overwhelming disease
B. Loss of potency of the antigen
C. Sarcoidosis
D. Hodgkin's disease
E. Steroids

Ref. N Engl J Med
285:1506, December 30, 1971

FOR EACH OF THE FOLLOWING QUESTIONS, SELECT THE ONE APPROPRIATE ANSWER BY USING THE KEY OUTLINED BELOW:

1. If A, B and C are correct
2. If A and C are correct
3. If B and D are correct
4. If all are correct
5. If all are incorrect

BRONCHIOLITIS

677. IN ASSESSING A POSSIBLE ATOPIC COMPONENT IN INFANTS WITH THE BRONCHIOLITIS SYNDROME, WHICH OF THE FOLLOWING MAY BE HELPFUL?:

A. Family history
B. Elevations of serum IgE
C. Recurrent attacks and previous eczema
D. Positive virus serology
E. Intracutaneous and provocation tests

Ref. Acta Paediat Scand
60:621, 1971

CYSTS, BRONCHOGENIC

678. CLINICAL DIFFERENTIATION BETWEEN ACQUIRED AND CONGENITAL PULMONARY CYSTS MAY BE DIFFICULT OR IMPOSSIBLE. WHICH OF THE FOLLOWING CHARACTERIZE BRONCHOGENIC CYSTS?:

A. Usually present as mediastinal masses
B. Typically, are unilocular and fluid-filled
C. Do not communicate with the tracheobronchial tree
D. Frequently, are asymptomatic
E. Symptoms are usually secondary to compression of adjacent pulmonary structures

Ref. J Pediatr Surg
6:255, June, 1971

IODIDES AND CYSTIC FIBROSIS

679. ALTHOUGH THE EFFICACY OF IODIDES IN INFLUENCING BRONCHIAL SECRETIONS IS QUESTIONED, THEIR CHRONIC ADMINISTRATION TO PATIENTS WITH CYSTIC FIBROSIS HAS BEEN ASSOCIATED WITH WHICH OF THE FOLLOWING SUSPECTED SIDE EFFECTS?:

A. Goiter
B. Nasal polyps
C. Hypothyroidism
D. Acne
E. Excessive lacrimation

Ref. J Pediatr
79:684, October, 1971

LUNG PUNCTURE

680. WHICH OF THE FOLLOWING FINDINGS HAVE BEEN DEMONSTRATED WITH THE USE OF LUNG PUNCTURE IN THE ETIOLOGICAL DIAGNOSIS OF PNEUMONIA IN INFANTS?:
A. Complications of needle aspiration of the lung should be infrequent
B. Lung puncture is the best available method for accurate etiologic diagnosis of pneumonias of infancy and childhood
C. The upper respiratory tract flora does not accurately represent the pathogenic flora in the lung
D. Opportunistic organisms have been isolated frequently from the lungs of malnourished children with pneumonia
E. Transient hemoptysis may follow diagnostic lung puncture

Ref. Am J Dis Child
122:278, October, 1971

681. LUNG PUNCTURE AND ASPIRATION HAS BEEN USEFUL IN INFANTS AND CHILDREN FOR THE IDENTIFICATION OF WHICH OF THE FOLLOWING CLINICAL AND INFLAMMATORY CONDITIONS?:
A. Pulmonary hemosiderosis
B. Pneumocystis carinii
C. Pseudomonas aeruginosa
D. Mycoplasma pneumoniae
E. Staphylococcus aureus

Ref. Am J Dis Child
122:278, October, 1971

PNEUMONIA, ADENOVIRUS

682. GASTROENTERITIS AND RASH ARE NOTED OFTEN IN CHILDREN WITH ADENOVIRUS INFECTIONS, BUT PNEUMONIA ASSOCIATED WITH TYPES 2, 3, 7 AND 21 ADENOVIRUSES IS A SEVERE DISEASE FOR INFANTS AND IS ACCOMPANIED OR FOLLOWED BY WHICH OF THE FOLLOWING?:
A. Obliterative bronchiolitis
B. Bronchiectasis
C. Pulmonary fibrosis
D. Pleural reactions
E. Bilateral infiltrations in majority

Ref. J Pediatr
79:605, October, 1971

FOR EACH OF THE FOLLOWING MULTIPLE CHOICE QUESTIONS, SELECT THE ONE MOST APPROPRIATE ANSWER:

ACETAMINOPHEN, PHENACETIN AND ACETANILID

683. IDENTIFY THE INCORRECT STATEMENT CONCERNING THE ANILINE DERIVATIVES (ACETAMINOPHEN, PHENACETIN AND ACETANILID) WHICH HAVE BEEN USED AS ANTIPYRETICS AND ANALGETICS:

A. "Phenacetin nephritis" remains largely unproven
B. Acetaminophen (Tylenol) has not been implicated in gastrointestinal bleeding
C. Acetanilid has been abondoned because of its association with methemoglobinemia and hemolytic anemia
D. Acetaminophen appears to be the analgetic equivalent to aspirin
E. Acetaminophen has been associated with hemolytic anemia in persons with glucose-6-phosphate dehydrogenase deficiency

Ref. N Engl J Med
286:20, January 6, 1972

ALIMENTATION, INTRAVENOUS

684. PEDIATRICIANS CARING FOR SICK CHILDREN WITH LONG-TERM NUTRITIONAL PROBLEMS SHOULD BE FAMILIAR WITH INTRAVENOUS ALIMENTATION. STANDARD RECOMMENDATIONS AND EXPERIENCE HAVE INCLUDED ALL OF THE FOLLOWING, EXCEPT:

A. An infusion pump aids in preventing plugging by thrombosis since reflux of blood into the catheter is prevented
B. The most common complication of intravenous alimentation is infection
C. Following insertion of the catheter its position should be confirmed by X-ray
D. Prophylactic antibiotics have decreased the incidence of infection
E. The inferior vena cava is prone to thrombosis when infused with hypertonic solutions

Ref. Pediatr Digest
13:30, April, 1971

ANTICONVULSANT THERAPY

685. IN THE SUCCESSFUL CONTROL OF EPILEPTIC SEIZURES IN CHILDREN ONE SHOULD OBSERVE ALL OF THE FOLLOWING PRINCIPLES, EXCEPT:

A. The longer epileptic seizures are permitted to go uncontrolled the less successful is their management and control
B. Diphenylhydantoin sodium (Dilantin) may increase the frequency of petit mal seizures
C. Hyperactivity simulating the hyperkinetic syndrome may appear in children during phenobarbital therapy
D. Anticonvulsant therapy may be discontinued in most girls at the onset of puberty
E. The dosage of anticonvulsant drugs, particularly phenobarbital, should be reduced very gradually because of the risk of recurrence of seizures and status epilepticus

Ref. Consultant
11:41, May, 1971

ANTIBIOTICS, FIXED DOSE COMBINATIONS

686. POSSIBLE REASONS FOR THE SIMULTANEOUS USE OF TWO OR MORE ANTIBIOTICS INCLUDE ALL OF THE FOLLOWING, EXCEPT:

A. Neonatal sepsis of unknown etiology
B. Mixed infections of the cardiovascular, respiratory or urinary systems
C. To delay the emergence of bacterial resistance to one drug, as in tuberculosis
D. "Synergism" that results from drug combinations is an established principle which can be utilized commonly in clinical infections
E. In some instances, two or more drugs used in combination may each be used in smaller doses than would be necessary if only one drug were used

Ref. JAMA
213:1172, August 17, 1970

ASPIRIN

687. ASPIRIN IS ASSOCIATED WITH ONE OUT OF FIVE CASES OF ACCIDENTAL POISONING. ALL OF THE FOLLOWING SIDE EFFECTS OF ASPIRIN HAVE BEEN OBSERVED IN CHILDREN, EXCEPT:

A. Thrombocytopenia
B. Asthma
C. Gastric ulceration
D. Low platelet ascorbic acid concentrations
E. Inhibition of prostaglandin synthesis

Ref. Infect Dis
1:3, August, 1971

ASPIRIN AND HEMOSTATIC MECHANISMS

688. CLINICAL AND EXPERIMENTAL EVIDENCE SUGGESTS THAT ASPIRIN PROFOUNDLY AFFECTS THE HEMOSTATIC MECHANISMS. EACH OF THE FOLLOWING STATEMENTS IS CORRECT, EXCEPT:

A. Aspirin causes occult gastrointestinal bleeding in most normal subjects
B. Aspirin given in large doses for several days can prolong the prothrombin time
C. Aggregation of platelets is impaired by aspirin
D. Platelet damage from aspirin is permanent for its life span
E. Acetaminophen has caused deleterious effects in hemostasis in both hemophiliacs and normal subjects

Ref. Mayo Clin Proc
46:178, March, 1971

BURNS AND SILVER NITRATE THERAPY

689. SILVER NITRATE DRESSINGS SHOULD BE APPLIED TO BURN WOUNDS IMMEDIATELY AFTER CLEANSING OF GREASE AND DIRT. ALL OF THE FOLLOWING ARE CORRECT IN REGARD TO SILVER NITRATE THERAPY, EXCEPT:

A. Silver nitrate is effective against both gram-negative and gram-positive bacteria
B. Eschar separation is accelerated
C. The patient and his environment assume a charcoal gray-brown hue
D. Occasional strains of Klebsiella and Proteus are capable of converting the nitrate to nitrite, thereby resulting in the formation of methemoglobin
E. Silver nitrate therapy contributes to sodium depletion

Ref. Infect Dis
1:9, May, 1971

BURNS AND SULFAMYLON

690. SYSTEMIC ABSORPTION FROM THE TOPICAL APPLICATION IN BURN THERAPY WITH MAFENIDE ACETATE (SULFAMYLON) HAS LED TO ALL OF THE FOLLOWING OBSERVATIONS, EXCEPT:

A. Peak blood levels occur within two to four hours of application
B. Decreased potassium excretion because of carbonic anhydrase inhibition
C. Normal or slightly elevated blood pH
D. Increased renal excretion of bicarbonate
E. Decreased arterial PCO_2

Ref. N Engl J Med 284:1281, June 10, 1971

CEPHALEXIN AND UREMIA

691. THE TREATMENT OF URINARY TRACT INFECTIONS CAUSED BY SUSCEPTIBLE ORGANISMS IN UREMIC PATIENTS IS COMPLICATED BY THE LIMITATIONS IMPOSED BY REDUCED RENAL FUNCTION WHICH INFLUENCES THE CONCENTRATION OF A GIVEN DRUG IN URINE. THE MARGIN OF SAFETY IN TREATING SUCH PROBLEMS APPEARS GREATEST WITH:

A. Oral cephalexin
B. Nitrofurantoin
C. Chloramphenicol
D. Kanamycin
E. Polymyxins

Ref. Ann Intern Med 72:349, March, 1970

CORTICOSTEROID THERAPY

692. PROLONGED SYSTEMIC CORTICOSTEROID THERAPY MAY BE ACCOMPANIED BY ALL OF THE FOLLOWING CLINICAL COMPLICATIONS AND LABORATORY FINDINGS, EXCEPT:

A. Centripetal fat deposition in the trunk, face and neck
B. Posterior subcapsular cataracts
C. Mediastinal lipomatosis with widening of the paraspinal tissues by X-ray
D. A decrease in the number of polymorphonuclear neutrophils
E. An elevation of the hemoglobin level without an increase in the number of erythrocytes

Ref. N Engl J Med 284:1357, June 17, 1971

DIAZEPAM IN HEROIN ADDICTION

693. MANAGEMENT OF ACUTE PHYSIOLOGIC WITHDRAWAL IN HEROIN ADDICTION IS AN INCREASING PROBLEM OF DRUG ABUSE IN ADOLESCENTS. EACH OF THE FOLLOWING IS CORRECT, EXCEPT:

A. Diarrhea is a common withdrawal symptom
B. Diazepam (Valium) appears to be effective in reducing the duration and severity of withdrawal symptoms
C. Yawning, lacrimation and "goose flesh" are common signs in heroin withdrawal
D. The physiologic disturbances of heroin withdrawal in humans persist for 48 to 72 hours
E. Insomnia is seen commonly in the withdrawal period

Ref. J Pediatr 78:692, April, 1971

DROWNING

694. THE PEDIATRICIAN IS OFTEN CONFRONTED WITH THE EMERGENCY TREATMENT OF CHILDREN WHO HAVE SUFFERED FROM NEAR DROWNING ACCIDENTS. EACH OF THE FOLLOWING STATEMENTS IN REGARD TO DROWNING IS CORRECT, EXCEPT:

A. Methylprednisolone has been shown to improve the mortality by improving oxygenation and ventilation
B. Near drowning in fresh water results in dry lungs
C. Patients die of progressive hypoxemia and respiratory acidosis
D. Hemodilution and hemolysis are risks in fresh water aspiration
E. Gross hemorrhage occurs in the lungs of rats after instillation of sea water

Ref. JAMA 215:1793, March 15, 1971

DRUGS AND BREAST FEEDING

695. WE KNOW LITTLE MORE TODAY ABOUT THE EFFECTS OF DRUGS TRANSMITTED TO THE INFANT THROUGH THE MOTHER'S BREAST THAN WE KNEW ABOUT DRUGS PASSING THROUGH THE PLACENTA BEFORE THE THALIDOMIDE INCIDENT. YOU WOULD BE INCLINED TO ADVISE AGAINST THE USE OF ALL OF THE FOLLOWING DRUGS WHILE BREAST-FEEDING, EXCEPT:

A. Salicylates
B. Steroids
C. Anticoagulants
D. Antithyroid drugs
E. Radioactive preparations

Ref. Nutrition Today 5:2, Winter, 1970

DRUGS AND CHROMOSOMAL BREAKAGE

696. ILLICIT DRUG USAGE HAS BECOME A SERIOUS MEDICAL AND SOCIAL PROBLEM. CONGENITAL MALFORMATIONS DUE TO CHROMOSOMAL BREAKAGE IN INFANTS BORN TO DRUG USERS HAVE BEEN ASSOCIATED WITH WHICH OF THE FOLLOWING AGENTS?:

A. LSD
B. STP
C. Heroin
D. Marijuana
E. None of the above

Ref. Pediatrics 47:1037, June, 1971

ENEMAS, SOAP

697. SOAP ENEMAS MAY BE HAZARDOUS AND ARE OF QUESTIONABLE VALUE. ALL OF THE FOLLOWING HAVE BEEN OBSERVED AS COMPLICATIONS OF THIS THERAPY, EXCEPT:

A. Hyperosmolar diarrhea
B. Proctitis
C. Rectal gangrene
D. Anaphylaxis
E. Acute soap colitis

Ref. N Engl J Med 285:217, July 22, 1971

GENTAMICIN AND SEPSIS

698. IN THE MANAGEMENT OF BACTERIAL SEPSIS DUE TO GRAM-NEGATIVE ORGANISMS IN THE YOUNG INFANT AND CHILD, ALL OF THE FOLLOWING ARE ACCEPTED AS THERAPEUTICALLY SOUND, EXCEPT:

A. During the first week of life, urinary excretion of gentamicin is slow, which prolongs the half-life in blood for five hours
B. The levels of gentamicin obtained in spinal fluid in newborn infants is high
C. Gentamicin is the drug of choice in sepsis due to Klebsiella and Pseudomonas
D. The cardiovascular management which includes maintenance of blood pressure and renal perfusion, is more important than the choice of an antibiotic, so long as the one selected is active in vitro against the organisms causing sepsis
E. Steroids contribute to survival from sepsis, particularly in maintaining blood pressure

Ref. Clin Pediatr
10:369, July, 1971

HEROIN AND ACUTE MYOGLOBINURIA

699. ACUTE RHABDOMYOLYSIS HAS BEEN OBSERVED AS A NEW COMPLICATION OF INTRAVENOUS HEROIN-ADULTERANT INJECTIONS. THE CLINICAL AND LABORATORY FEATURES WHICH HAVE ACCOMPANIED THE ACUTE SKELETAL NECROSIS HAVE INCLUDED ALL OF THE FOLLOWING, EXCEPT:

A. Acute myoglobinuria
B. Marked elevations of serum creatine phosphokinase
C. Renal failure
D. Generalized muscle tenderness and weakness
E. Irreversibility of clinical manifestations

Ref. JAMA
216:1172, May 17, 1971

HYDROCARBONS, CHLORINATED

700. ENVIRONMENTAL CONTAMINANTS, ESPECIALLY CHLORINATED HYDROCARBONS, HAVE LED TO MUCH SPECULATION AND ANXIETY-PROVOKING STATEMENTS. ALL OF THE FOLLOWING HAVE BEEN LABELED AS UNPROVED WITH THE EXCEPTION OF:

A. There has been no significant increase in the storage of DDT by the general population of the United States since it was first measured in 1950
B. DDT is carcinogenic to man
C. DDT significantly reduces photosynthesis in phytoplanktons
D. DDT as used at present influences human reproduction
E. DDT as used at the present time will control the population explosion, by destroying "all chlorophyl formers and hence all food supply," or by its effects on sex hormones

Ref. JAMA
212:1055, May 11, 1970

IMFERON AND PLEOCYTOSIS

701. THE INTRAMUSCULAR USE OF IRON DEXTRAN (IMFERON) HAS BEEN ASSOCIATED WITH ALL OF THE FOLLOWING REACTIONS, EXCEPT:

A. Fever
B. Jaundice
C. A leukemoid reaction
D. Pleocytosis
E. Arthralgia

Ref. Lancet
1:1428, 1968

LEAD POISONING

702. CHILDHOOD LEAD POISONING IS A MAJOR HEALTH PROBLEM. THE SYSTEMIC SCREENING OF SUSPECT POPULATIONS HAS BEEN RECOMMENDED. EACH OF THE FOLLOWING IS CORRECT CONCERNING LEAD POISONING, EXCEPT:

A. Red cell aminolevulinic acid dehydratase is a useful screening procedure for lead poisoning
B. A precise correlation between blood lead and subclinical and clinical disease has not been established
C. Urinary coproporphyrins are not uniformly positive in children with lead levels higher than 80 micrograms per 100 ml
D. Anemia and basophilic stippling are uniform and reliable laboratory findings in lead intoxication
E. Enzyme inhibition and disturbances in heme synthesis can be demonstrated at levels less than 60 micrograms suggesting that any degree of lead exposure is potentially harmful

Ref. N Engl J Med
284:565, March 18, 1971

LEAD

703. THE TOXIC EFFECTS ON BODY BIOCHEMISTRY OF LEAD APPEAR TO BE IN THE AREA OF HEME SYNTHESIS, CELLULAR RESPIRATION AND MEMBRANE FUNCTION. EACH OF THE FOLLOWING STATEMENTS IS CORRECT CONCERNING THIS MAJOR HEALTH HAZARD FOR CHILDREN, EXCEPT:

A. Blood lead levels in children do not rise rapidly from continued ingestion, and it is not accepted that levels of 40 to 60 micrograms per 100 ml could surpass 100 micrograms in a period of one to two months
B. Blood lead does not appear to be in equilibrium with the total body lead burden
C. Most of body lead is tightly bound in bone
D. "Mobile" pools of lead are located primarily in the soft tissues
E. Levels of 80 micrograms per 100 ml of blood suggest an unacceptable risk that demands immediate hospitalization for chelation therapy, regardless of the presence or absence of clinical symptoms

Ref. Pediatrics
48:349, September, 1971

LICORICE INTOXICATION

704. HABITUAL LICORICE INGESTION HAS LED TO ALL OF THE FOLLOWING, EXCEPT:
A. Metabolic alkalosis
B. Hypokalemia
C. An increase in aldosterone secretion and suppression of plasma renin
D. Hypertension
E. Sodium and water retention

Ref. Pennsylvania Med 74:51, March, 1971

MAGNESIUM

705. THE INTRAVENOUS ADMINISTRATION OF MAGNESIUM SULFATE TO A TOXEMIC MOTHER MAY HAVE PROFOUND CLINICAL AND BIOCHEMICAL EFFECTS ON THE NEWBORN INFANT. EACH OF THE FOLLOWING STATEMENTS IN REGARD TO NEONATAL HYPERMAGNESEMIA IS CORRECT, EXCEPT:
A. The newborn may require assisted ventilation and resuscitation as the result of respiratory depression and muscle weakness
B. Intravenous calcium given to compromised hypermagnesemic newborn infants has resulted in dramatic clinical improvement
C. Exchange transfusion may reverse the toxity of hypermagnesemia in the newborn
D. Forced diuresis does not appear to be a satisfactory method of treating these infants
E. When magnesium sulfate is given intramuscularly to the mother the newborn is usually not affected by excess magnesium

Ref. Pediatrics 47:501, 1971

MARIHUANA AND THE "SOCIAL HIGH"

706. RELATIVELY FEW STUDIES DEALING WITH THE EFFECTS OF MARIHUANA ON CEREBRAL FUNCTIONS ARE AVAILABLE. HOWEVER, EACH OF THE FOLLOWING PHENOMENA WAS OBSERVED IN A MARIHUANA-INDUCED "SOCIAL HIGH," EXCEPT:
A. There is a slight but statistically significant shift toward slower frequencies in the electroencephalogram
B. Bender-Gestalt drawings are executed more poorly after drug inhalation
C. Vibratory sense appreciation improves slightly
D. Ataxia and impairment of cortical sensation are common
E. There is no evidence of an increased tendency for illusion, hallucinations of delusional thinking

Ref. JAMA 213:1300, August 24, 1970

MERCURY

707. GREAT CONCERN OVER ENVIRONMENTAL CONTAMINATION FROM MERCURY WAS VOICED IN 1970-71. EACH OF THE FOLLOWING STATEMENTS IS CORRECT, EXCEPT:

A. The symptoms of organic mercury poisoning involve chiefly the central nervous system and may mimic encephalitis
B. In Japan several infants with increased exposure to mercury were born with congenital cerebral paresis to mothers who showed no signs of mercury intoxication during pregnancy
C. Enormous quantities of canned tuna were removed from the American market by the Food and Drug Administration but one could eat a 7 oz. can (containing 0.5 ppm) daily for years and expect mercury whole blood levels to remain within a safe range for non-pregnant adults
D. Apart from the risk to both prenatal and postnatal children the risk of organic mercury compounds in food has probably been overstated
E. The fetal and infant central nervous systems are far more resistant to mercury toxicity than the adult

Ref. N Engl J Med 284:706, April 1, 1971

HAZARDS OF LAUNDRY PRODUCTS

708. PHYSICIANS IN CHARGE OF NEWBORN NURSERIES SHOULD BE FAMILIAR WITH LAUNDERING PROCEDURES USED IN TREATING INFANT'S CLOTHING, BEDDING AND DIAPERS. METHEMOGLOBINEMIA HAS BEEN ASSOCIATED WITH THE PERCUTANEOUS ABSORPTION OF TRICHLOROCARBANILIDE (TCC) AND THE SODIUM SALT OF PENTACHLOROPHENOL (PCP) IN NEWBORNS. ALL OF THE FOLLOWING ARE CORRECT IN REGARD TO NEONATAL METHEMOGLOBINEMIA, EXCEPT:

A. Excessive doses of methylene blue in the treatment of methemoglobinemia in the newborn may damage the erythrocytes
B. The blood from infants with methemoglobinemia is chocolate brown in the test tube and does not turn red on shaking with air
C. Infants with methemoglobinemia demonstrate cyanosis with dyspnea when levels of methemoglobin exceed 10% of the total hemoglobin
D. The blood from a cyanotic and hypoxic infant will turn brighter red on exposure to air on a glass slide
E. Methemoglobinemia persisting in spite of methylene blue administration is suggestive of an abnormal methemoglobin M

Ref. Newsletter, Am Acad Pediatr 22:2, July 15, 1971

METHADONE

709. A 2 YEAR-OLD CHILD WITH RESPIRATORY DEPRESSION HAS BEEN ACCIDENTALLY POISONED WITH BARBITURATES, BUT IS THOUGHT TO HAVE INGESTED METHADONE. WHICH OF THE FOLLOWING INTRAVENOUS DRUGS USED IN THE TREATMENT OF RESPIRATORY DEPRESSION WILL NOT AGGRAVATE THE PROBLEM IN THIS YOUNGSTER?:

A. Naloxone hydrochloride (Narcan)
B. Nalorphine hydrochloride (Nalline)
C. Levallorphan tartrate (Lorfan)
D. All of the above
E. None of the above

Ref. Pediatrics 48:173, August, 1971

METHADONE AND CHILDREN

710. ACCIDENTAL METHADONE POISONING OF SMALL CHILDREN HAS BEEN REPORTED WITH INCREASING FREQUENCY IN LARGE URBAN CENTERS. THE TREATMENT OF CHOICE APPEARS TO BE:

A. Naloxone hydrochloride (Narcan)
B. Thorazine
C. Exchange transfusion
D. Dialysis
E. Central nervous system stimulants

Ref. Pediatrics
48:173, August, 1971

METHADONE INTOXICATION

711. THE NEUROPHYSIOLOGIC EFFECTS OF METHADONE, WITH FEW EXCEPTIONS, ARE MOST COMPARABLE TO THOSE OF MORPHINE. WHICH OF THE FOLLOWING COMPLICATIONS OF ACCIDENTAL METHADONE POISONING HAS BEEN DESCRIBED FOR THE FIRST TIME IN A CHILD?:

A. Pulmonary edema
B. Orthostatic hypotension
C. Urinary retention
D. Elevated cerebral spinal fluid pressure
E. Respiratory depression

Ref. Pediatrics
48:294, August, 1971

ORGANOPHOSPHATES

712. THE ORGANOPHOSPHATES (PARATHION, MALATHION,ETC.) ARE THE PESTICIDES MOST OFTEN INVOLVED IN SERIOUS POISONING IN CHILDREN, AND WITH RECENT GOVERNMENT REGULATIONS AGAINST THE USE OF DDT THE INCIDENCE OF POISONING WITH THESE AGENTS MAY WELL INCREASE. ALL OF THE FOLLOWING ARE CHARACTERISTIC OF THIS CLASS OF PESTICIDES, EXCEPT:

A. All are cholinesterase inhibitors
B. All penetrate the intact skin
C. There is no accumulation in the body
D. Confirmation of poisoning is based on depression of plasma and red blood cell cholinesterase, and no treatment should be instituted until this determination is made
E. Organophosphates are nonpersistent in the environment

Ref. JAMA
216:2131, June 28, 1971

713. IN PARATHION POISONING (ORGANOPHOSPHATE) WHICH OF THE FOLLOWING DRUGS AIDS IN THE REGENERATION OF CHOLINESTERASE AND REVERSAL OF MUSCLE WEAKNESS WHICH MAY BE RESPONSIBLE FOR RESPIRATORY EMBARRASSMENT AND POSSIBLE DEATH?:

A. Atropine
B. Pralidoxime (Protopam) chloride
C. Morphine
D. Aminophylline
E. Phenothiazines

Ref. JAMA
216:2131, June 28, 1971

PHARMACOGENETICS

714. GENETIC DIFFERENCES IN THE METABOLISM OF DRUGS ARE WIDESPREAD, AND PHARMACOGENETICS UNDERLIES MANY ANOMALOUS DRUG RESPONSES. EACH OF THE FOLLOWING IS CORRECT, EXCEPT:

A. Children with the Crigler-Najjar syndrome are abnormally sensitive to salicylates
B. Individuals with Down's syndrome are hypersensitive to atropine
C. Sulfonamides may induce methemoglobinemia and a fulminating hemolytic anemia in patients with Zurich hemoglobin
D. The sickle-cell trait gives a degree of protection to the heterozygote against malignant falciparum malaria
E. All variants of the enzyme defect involving glucose-6-phosphate dehydrogenase (which affects some tens of millions of people) are drug sensitive to such agents as primaquine, sulfonamides and para-amino salicylic acid

Ref. Hospital Pract 6:97, June, 1971

PHARMACOGENETICS

715. A PEDIATRICIAN SHOULD CONSIDER THE POSSIBILITY OF AN INHERITED DRUG ANOMALY WHENEVER INEXPLICABLE REACTIONS OCCUR TO MEDICATIONS. EACH OF THE FOLLOWING IS CORRECT, EXCEPT:

A. Coumarin anticoagulant resistance is an example of a receptor site disorder where a normal dose of a drug fails to achieve the desired response
B. Hemoglobin Zurich and favism are examples of tissue metabolism disorders in which a normal dose of a drug produces a normal blood level but the patient "overreacts" because his tissues or red cells are peculiarly vulnerable to the drug
C. Extensive studies have shown no variations in the metabolism of isoniazid amongst individuals which have included identical and fraternal twins
D. Isoniazid can produce diphenylhydantoin (Dilantin) sensitivity when the two drugs are given together
E. Slow inactivators of succinylcholine are examples of drug metabolism disorders in which a normal dose of a drug will produce an abnormally high blood level

Ref. Hospital Pract 6:105, June, 1971

PHOTOTOXICITY

716. PHOTOTOXIC REACTIONS MAY BE INDUCED AFTER ORAL, PARENTERAL OR EXTERNAL CONTACT WITH DRUGS. ALL OF THE FOLLOWING ANTIFUNGAL AND ANTIBACTERIAL AGENTS HAVE BEEN ASSOCIATED WITH PHOTOTOXICITY, EXCEPT:

A. Tetracyclines
B. Rifampin
C. Sulfonamides
D. Griseofulvin
E. Nalidixic acid

Ref. JAMA 217:1091, August 23, 1971

PROPOXYPHENE (DARVON)

717. ALTHOUGH WIDELY USED AS AN ANALGESIC, ALL OF THE FOLLOWING ARE CORRECT IN REGARD TO THE USE OF PROPOXYPHENE (DARVON), EXCEPT:
A. Propoxyphene is related structurally to methadone
B. 32 mg by mouth has little more than placebo effect on pain
C. 65 to 100 mg by mouth is inferior to aspirin or codeine in analgetic efficacy
D. The addiction potential of propoxyphene is comparable to the opioids
E. Nalorphine is effective in combating the respiratory depression associated with intoxication

Ref. N Engl J Med
286:20, January 6, 1972

RIFAMPIN

718. ALL OF THE FOLLOWING ARE IN ACCORDANCE WITH THE RECOMMENDATIONS FOR LABELING OF RIFAMPIN, EXCEPT:
A. Rifampin is not indicated in the treatment of meningococcal infections
B. The drug should be used in the treatment of asymptomic meningococcal carriers in situations in which the risk of secondary cases is high
C. Rifampin should not be used as the sole therapeutic agent for the initial treatment of pulmonary tuberculosis
D. Periodic liver function monitoring is suggested during long-term therapy with Rifampin
E. In the retreatment of patients with pulmonary tuberculosis the use of Rifampin compares favorably with the combination of Rifampin and isoniazid in producing negative sputum cultures

Ref. Med Tribune
12:3, June 16, 1971

SALICYLATE DISTRIBUTION AND pH

719. IN EXPERIMENTAL SALICYLATE POISONING IMPORTANT OBSERVATIONS HAVE BEEN MADE ON THE EFFECTS OF ALTERING BLOOD pH ON TISSUE AND PLASMA SALICYLATE CONCENTRATIONS. ALL OF THE FOLLOWING HAVE BEEN OBSERVED, EXCEPT:
A. Bicarbonate infusions in experimental salicylate poisoning raise blood pH and lower muscle, brain and liver salicylate concentrations compared with controls
B. Mortality in salicylate poisoning is not associated with salicylate levels in the brain of animals
C. Carbon dioxide inhalation produces a shift of salicylate into the tissues and out of the plasma
D. Acetazolamide lowers blood pH, raises the tissue salicylate levels and increases the toxicity of sodium salicylate
E. If the systemic acidosis produced by acetazolamide is prevented with bicarbonate, the rise in tissue salicylate is also prevented

Ref. Pediatrics
47:658, 1971

SUBCLAVIAN PUNCTURES

720. THE SUBCLAVIAN ROUTE FOR THE "BLIND" PLACEMENT OF A CENTRAL VENOUS CATHETER HAS BEEN MOST COMMONLY ASSOCIATED WITH WHICH OF THE FOLLOWING COMPLICATIONS?:

A. Pneumothorax
B. Laceration of the subclavian artery
C. Subclavian vein thrombosis
D. Fatal air embolism
E. Penetration of the right atrium with cardiac tamponade

Ref. JAMA
217:78, July 5, 1971

VALIUM

721. VALIUM (DIAZEPAM) IS USED WIDELY IN THE CONTROL OF CONVULSIONS AND AS A RELAXANT FOR INFANTS ON RESPIRATORY CARE. THE INJECTABLE FORM CONTAINS 5 PER CENT SODIUM BENZOATE AND BENZOIC ACID AS BUFFERS AND SHOULD BE USED WITH CAUTION OR NOT AT ALL IN NEONATES WITH ELEVATED SERUM BILIRUBIN LEVELS BECAUSE:

A. The dose has not been determined
B. It is usually ineffective in the control of seizures in this age group
C. The possibility of hepatotoxicity
D. It is a potent bilirubin-albumin uncoupler
E. The risk of hemolysis in glucose-6-PD deficient red cells

Ref. Pediatrics
48:139, July, 1971

FOR EACH OF THE FOLLOWING QUESTIONS, SELECT THE ONE APPROPRIATE ANSWER BY USING THE KEY OUTLINED BELOW:

1. If A, B and C are correct
2. If A and C are correct
3. If B and D are correct
4. If all are correct
5. If all are incorrect

AMINOPHYLINE

722. AMINOPHYLINE HAS A SIGNIFICANT THERAPEUTIC EFFECT IN STATUS ASTHMATICUS BUT MAY BE ASSOCIATED WITH WHICH OF THE FOLLOWING TOXIC REACTIONS?:

A. Gastrointestinal bleeding
B. Cardiac arrhythmias
C. Shock
D. Delirium
E. Convulsions

Ref. Pediatrics
48:642, October, 1971

ANALGESICS AND ADDICTION

723. WHICH OF THE FOLLOWING ANALGETIC DRUGS ARE NON-ADDICTING?:
A. Methadone
B. Methotrimeprazine (Levoprome)
C. Pentazocine (Talwin)
D. Nalorphine (Nalline)
E. Meperidine (Demerol)

Ref. N Engl J Med
286:249, February 3, 1972

DIPHENYLHYDANTION

724. WHICH OF THE FOLLOWING DRUGS HAVE BEEN ASSOCIATED WITH SOURCES OF ERROR IN THE DETERMINATION OF DIPHENYLHYDANTOIN (DILANTIN) LEVELS IN SERUM?:
A. Ethosuximide (Zarontin)
B. Mephenytoin (Mesantoin)
C. Phenylbutazone (Butazolidin)
D. Primidone
E. Teething lotion (Oil of cloves, oil of sassafrass)

Ref. Am J Dis Child
122:259, September, 1971

HEXACHLOROPHENE

725. HEXACHLOROPHENE IS AN INGRDIENT OF SOME 300 TO 400 PRODUCTS AND INCLUDED IN ITS MOST NEEDLESS USES IS IN VAGINAL DEODORANTS, WHICH HAS BEEN CALLED A $53 MILLION-A-YEAR RACKET. HEXACHLOROPHENE HAS BEEN ASSOCIATED WITH WHICH OF THE FOLLOWING?:
A. Small concentrations have produced brain damage in rats
B. Burn encephalopathies
C. Chloasma
D. Significant absorption from the skins of newborn infants
E. Significant absorption from its incorporation in mouthwashes

Ref. Science
174:805, November, 1971

LEAD

726. THE UNITED STATES PUBLIC HEALTH SERVICE HAS SUGGESTED THAT WHEN LABORATORY FACILITIES ARE LIMITED FOR MAKING A DIAGNOSIS OF LEAD POISONING THAT CERTAIN OF THE FOLLOWING MAY BE CONSIDERED INDICATIVE OF LEAD INTOXICATION:
A. Basophilic stippling of red blood cells
B. "Lead lines" in long bone X-rays
C. Strongly positive urine spot test for coproporphyrin
D. Hemoglobin of less than 10 grams
E. X-ray of the abdomen

Ref. Pediatrics
48:464, September, 1971

LEAD AND DEVELOPMENTAL STATUS

727. A CONTROLLED STUDY OF THE DEVELOPMENT OF CHILDREN WITH ELEVATED BLOOD LEAD LEVELS DEMONSTRATED WHICH OF THE FOLLOWING?:

A. Higher incidence of deficiencies of fine motor function in lead group
B. Higher correlation of developmental delays with the quality of mother-child relationships
C. Increased delays in language development in children with elevated lead levels
D. No significant differences in developmental scores between the lead and control groups
E. Direct correlation of developmental problems with lead levels

Ref. J Pediatr
80:57, January, 1972

IMIPRAMINE INTOXICATION

728. IMIPRAMINE HYDROCHLORIDE (TOFRANIL) IS USED WIDELY BY PEDIATRICIANS IN THE TREATMENT OF ENURESIS AND HAS BEEN ASSOCIATED WITH WHICH OF THE FOLLOWING REACTIONS?:

A. Electrocardiographic abnormalities
B. Fatalities from accidental ingestion
C. Postural hypotension
D. Extrapyramidal neurologic symptoms
E. Excessive sweating

Ref. Pediatrics
48:777, November, 1971
Pediatrics
47:132, January, 1071

IRON POISONING

729. A PLAN FOR THE TREATMENT OF ACCIDENTAL IRON INGESTION SHOULD BE FLEXIBLE BUT SHOULD INCLUDE WHICH OF THE FOLLOWING IN CHILDREN WHO PRESENT WITHOUT SHOCK OR COMA?:

A. Gastric lavage with half-strength Fleet's enema (sodium dihydrogen phosphate)
B. Deferoxamine therapy should be started when the serum iron level is in excess of the total iron binding capacity
C. Serum iron levels that remain below the total iron binding capacity four to five hours after ingestions probably do not require chelation therapy
D. If the above laboratory determinations cannot be obtained rapidly, treatment should be instituted if the ingested elemental iron is greater than 500 mgm
E. Blood pressure monitoring during deferoxamine therapy

Ref. JAMA
218:1179, November 22, 1971

METHOTREXATE

730. METHOTREXATE IS A SYNTHETIC ANTIMETABOLITE OF FOLIC ACID WHICH INHIBITS THE SYNTHESIS OF DEOXYRIBONUCELIC ACID (DNA) AND HAS BEEN ASSOCIATED WITH WHICH OF THE FOLLOWING TOXICITIES?:

A. Hepatic fibrosis
B. Megaloblastic anemia
C. Alopecia
D. Suppression of hematopoiesis
E. Granulomatous pneumonitis

Ref. Br Med J
4:467, November 20, 1971

PENICILLIN AND SKIN RASHES

731. THE OCCURRENCE OF RASH IN ASSOCIATION WITH PENICILLIN THERAPY IS A COMMON CLINICAL EVENT, AND ONE WHICH OFTEN POSES A THERAPEUTIC DILEMMA. WHICH OF THE FOLLOWING ARE CORRECT?:

A. A positive skin test to penicilloyl-polylysine (PPL) or to the minor determinant mixture (MDM) is strong evidence implicating penicillin as causing an urticarial rash
B. In the majority of ampicillin-associated morbilliform rashes, no unusual immune response has been detected
C. Current data indicate that with negative skin tests to PPL and MDM, patients can receive penicillin without anticipating an immediate or anaphylactic reaction
D. Cephalosporins may be safely substituted in penicillin allergic children
E. Skin testing with PPL and MDM may be done on appearance of the rash, and need not be repeated if negative

Ref. N Engl J Med
286:42, January 6, 1972

PHENYLBUTAZONE (BUTAZOLIDIN)

732. PHENYLBUTAZONE (BUTAZOLIDIN) HAS SERIOUS ADVERSE EFFECTS WHICH INCLUDE WHICH OF THE FOLLOWING?:

A. Aganulocytosis
B. Thrombocytopenia
C. Aplastic anemia
D. Hepatitis
E. Pepetic ulceration

Ref. N Engl J Med
286:20, January 6, 1972

PIPERAZINE NEUROTOXICITY: "WORM WOBBLE"

733. PIPERAZINE CITRATE IS WIDELY USED IN THE TREATMENT OF PINWORMS AND HAS PROVOKED WHICH OF THE FOLLOWING NEUROLOGIC SIGNS?:

A. Hypotonia
B. Cerebellar ataxia
C. Blurred vision
D. Deafness
E. Sensory neuropathies

Ref. Br Med J
4:792, December 25, 1971

RIFAMPIN AND TOXICITY

734. RIFAMPICIN IS A VALUABLE DRUG WITH GREAT EFFECTIVENESS AND LOW TOXICITY WHEN USED ON A DAILY BASIS AT RECOMMENDED DOSES. HOWEVER, WHICH OF THE FOLLOWING SIDE REACTIONS WERE NOTED IN PATIENTS WHEN TWICE-WEEKLY HIGH DOSES WERE USED IN THE TREATMENT OF TUBERCULOSIS?:

A. Fever
B. Thrombocytopenia
C. Jaundice
D. Coombs' positive hemolytic anemia
E. Gastrointestinal bleeding

Ref. Br Med J
3:343, August 7, 1971

CHELATING AGENTS

FOR THE FOLLOWING MATCHING QUESTIONS, CHOOSE THE ONE STATEMENT IN THE RIGHT HAND COLUMN WHICH BEST APPLIES TO THE STATEMENT IN THE LEFT HAND COLUMN. STATEMENTS ON THE RIGHT MAY BE USED MORE THAN ONCE:

735. ___ Pyridoxine antagonist
736. ___ Hypocalcemia
737. ___ Lacrimation and salivation
738. ___ Nephrotic syndrome

A. Dimercaprol (BAL)
B. EDTA
C. Desferrioxamine B
D. Penicillamine

Ref. Br Med J
2:270, May 1, 1971

DRUG COMBINATIONS

OF THE 200 MOST FREQUENTLY PRESCRIBED DRUGS IN 1970, A TOTAL OF 78 WERE FIXED DRUG COMBINATIONS. PHYSICIANS PRESCRIBE COMBINATION DRUGS IN TWO OUT OF EVERY FIVE PRESCRIPTIONS THEY WRITE. MATCH THE COMBINATIONS WITH THEIR COMPONENTS IN THE FOLLOWING COMMONLY PRESCRIBED DRUGS:

A. Achrocidin tablets
B. Actifed
C. Benylin expectorant
D. Dimetapp
E. Lomotil
F. Mycolog
G. Mysteclin F
H. Ornade

739. ___ Triprolidine HCL, pseudoephedrine HCL
740. ___ Tetracycline HCL, phenacetin, caffeine, salicylamide, chlorothen citrate
741. ___ Triamcinolone acetonide, neomycin sulfate, gramicidin, nystatin
742. ___ Diphenhydramine HCL, ammonium chloride, sodium citrate, chloroform
743. ___ Chlorpheniramine maleate, phenylpropanolamine HCL, isopropamideiodide
744. ___ Brompheniramine maleate, phenylphrine HCL, phenylpropanolamine HCL
745. ___ Atropine sulfate, diphenoxylate HCL
746. ___ Tetracycline, amphotericin B., potassium metaphosphate

Ref. JAMA
216:1009, May 10, 1971

FOR EACH OF THE FOLLOWING MULTIPLE CHOICE QUESTIONS, SELECT THE ONE APPROPRIATE ANSWER:

BREAST MILK AND CANCER

747. SIMILARITIES BETWEEN ADENOCARCINOMA OF THE BREAST IN MICE AND WOMEN ARE TOO EXTENSIVE TO BE COINCIDENCE, AND IT IS POSSIBLE THAT HUMAN BREAST CANCER MAY ALSO BE A VIRUS INDUCED DISEASE. EACH OF THE FOLLOWING OBSERVATIONS ARE CORRECT, EXCEPT:

A. In countries in which prolonged breast feeding is customary cancer of the breast is rare
B. Virus particles which are identical with the Bittner virus (associated with mammary adenocarcinoma in mice) have been found in the milk of humans
C. The virus is transmitted usually from mother to offspring (mice) in milk rather than through the placenta
D. Virus particles have been found in the milk of women with a family history of breast carcinoma with higher frequency than in the milk of controls
E. Evidence for horizontal transmission of breast cancer in mice suggests the possibility of a contagious component other than in milk

Ref. Nature 229:611, February 26, 1971

CARCINOMA, MEDULLARY OF THYROID

748. MEDULLARY CARCINOMA OF THE THYROID MAY ACCOUNT FOR 5 TO 10 PER CENT OF ALL THYROID CARCINOMAS AND WAS FIRST DESCRIBED AS A CLINICOPATHOLOGIC ENTITY IN 1959. THE NEWER CLINICAL FEATURES WHICH HAVE BEEN DISCOVERED HAVE INCLUDED ALL OF THE FOLLOWING, EXCEPT:

A. Association with other tumors such as pheochromocytoma, parathyroid adenoma and mucocutaneous neuromata
B. Severe unexplained diarrhea
C. Association with other syndromes and structural abnormalities including Cushing's syndrome, carcinoid syndrome, situs inversus and the Marfan's habitus
D. Familial incidence and autosomal dominant trait
E. Hashimoto's thyroiditis

Ref. N Engl J Med 283:890, October 22, 1970

EPSTEIN-BARR VIRUS

749. THE EPSTEIN-BARR VIRUS, A HERPES-LIKE AGENT, HAS BEEN ASSOCIATED WITH ALL OF THE FOLLOWING, EXCEPT:

A. Infectious mononucleosis
B. Nasopharyngeal carcinoma
C. Burkitt lymphoma
D. The stimulation of DNA production by infected lymphocytes from donors who are negative for EB virus antibody
E. Antibodies to the Epstein-Barr virus are rare in children living in low socioeconomic conditions

Ref. Hospital Pract 5:33, July, 1970

CHRONIC DIARRHEA WITH GANGLIONEUROBLASTOMA

750. NEUROGENIC TUMORS ARISING FROM THE GANGLION CELL SERIES SHOULD BE CONSIDERED IN THE CHILD WITH CHRONIC UNEXPLAINED DIARRHEA. ALL OF THE FOLLOWING ARE TRUE, EXCEPT:

A. The mechanism by which neurogenic tumors such as ganglioneuroblastoma produce diarrhea is not understood
B. Not all children with catecholamine secreting neurogenic tumors have diarrhea
C. Patients with pheochromocytomas do not usually have diarrhea
D. The absence of elevated urine levels of vanillylmandelic acid and catecholamines excludes a functioning neurogenic tumor
E. Diarrhea ceases after the complete removal of the neurogenic tumor

Ref. Clin Pediatr
10:476, August, 1971

ADENOCARCINOMA OF VAGINA

751. CLUSTERING OF MALIGNANCIES MAY SHED LIGHT ON ENVIRONMENTAL FACTORS IN CONGENITAL DISEASE. VAGINAL BLEEDING IN YOUNG WOMEN HAS BEEN ASSOCIATED WITH ADENOCARCINOMA OF THE VAGINA. WHICH OF THE FOLLOWING IS UNDER SUSPICION AS A POSSIBLE FACTOR IN THIS UNUSUAL TUMOR?:

A. Early sexual exposure
B. Administration of diethylstilbestrol to their mothers in the first trimester of pregnancy
C. History of tonsillectomy
D. Childhood ingestions
E. Intravaginal irritants (douches or tampons)

Ref. N Engl J Med
284:878, April 22, 1971

HISTIOCYTOSIS X, PULMONARY MANIFESTATIONS

752. THE PULMONARY MANIFESTATIONS OF HISTIOCYTOSIS X INCLUDE ALL OF THE FOLLOWING, EXCEPT:

A. Bilateral hilar node enlargement is an expected feature
B. Recurrent pneumothoraces
C. Apical bullae
D. Mottling, reticulation and honeycombing
E. Clearing of abnormal radiological signs may follow the use of corticosteroids

Ref. Proceedings Roy Soc Med
64:338, April, 1971

HODGKIN'S DISEASE

753. IN THE CLINICAL AND LABORATORY MANAGEMENT OF HODGKIN'S DISEASE ONE MIGHT EXPECT ALL OF THE FOLLOWING, EXCEPT:

A. A palpable spleen nearly always indicates involvement by Hodgkin's disease
B. There are no reported cases of Hodgkin's disease in the liver without concomitant involvement of the spleen which suggests that the pathway of spread to the liver may be by way of the spleen
C. Removal of the spleen reduces the radiation exposure to the left kidney
D. The mononucleosis spot test may be positive in Hodgkin's and non-Hodgkin's lymphomas
E. Reed-Sternberg cells have occasionally been found in lymph-node biopsy in cases of documented infectious mononucleosis

Ref. N Engl J Med
284:904 April 22, 1971

754. HODGKIN'S DISEASE HAS BEEN NOTED TO AFFECT DISPROPORTIONATELY THOSE IN BETTER SOCIO-ECONOMIC CONDITIONS. RECENTLY, EACH OF THE FOLLOWING HAS BEEN NOTED TO BE CORRECT, EXCEPT:

A. Cervical Hodgkin's disease frequently bypasses the mediastinum and may involve the spleen in the absence of splenomegaly
B. Extensive disease in the retroperitoneal nodes and spleen may be present in Hodgkin's disease although lymphangiography and inferior vena cavagraphy are negative
C. The chest is the most frequently involved body region in Hodgkin's
D. Tonsillectomy appears to increase the liability to the development of Hodgkin's disease
E. Hodgkin's disease, in contrast to other lymphomas, frequently involves the lymphoid tissues of Waldeyer's ring

Ref. Lancet
1:431, February, 1971

IMMUNOLOGY AND NEOPLASIA

755. EVIDENCE EXISTS THAT THE IMMUNE SYSTEM MAINTAINS SURVEILLANCE OF THE BODY TO DESTROY CONTINUALLY APPEARING POTENTIALLY MALIGNANT CELLS. AN INCREASED INCIDENCE OF MALIGNANT DISEASE HAS BEEN REPORTED IN ALL OF THE FOLLOWING CLINICAL OR EXPERIMENTAL MODELS, EXCEPT:

A. Prolonged treatment with immunosuppressive drugs
B. The use of antilymphocyte serum
C. Thymectomized newborn mice
D. Congenital cellular immune deficiency diseases
E. Chronic granulomatous disease

Ref. Clin Pediatr
10:373, July, 1971

SACROCOCCYGEAL MASSES

756. CALCIFICATION WITHIN A SKIN-COVERED SACROCOCCYGEAL MASS IN A NEWBORN INFANT IS HIGHLY SUGGESTIVE OF:

A. Teratoma
B. Lipomeningocele
C. Lipoma
D. Meningocele
E. "Mixed neural" (myelocystocele)

Ref. J Pediatr
79:948, December, 1971

THYMUS

757. IN LATE CHILDHOOD AN ENLARGED THYMUS MAY BE ASSOCIATED WITH ALL OF THE FOLLOWING, EXCEPT:

A. No disease
B. Corticosteroid administration
C. Thyrotoxicosis
D. Lymphomas
E. Myasthenia gravis

Ref. Radiology
101:625, December, 1971

FOR EACH OF THE FOLLOWING QUESTIONS, SELECT THE ONE MOST APPROPRIATE ANSWER BY USING THE KEY OUTLINED BELOW:

1. If A, B and C are correct
2. If A and C are correct
3. If B and D are correct
4. If all are correct
5. If all are incorrect

HEPATIC TUMORS

758. ANGIOGRAPHY IS DISTINCTIVE IN DIFFERENTIATING PRIMARY FROM SECONDARY TUMORS OF THE LIVER IN WHICH OF THE FOLLOWING CATEGORIES?:
A. Delayed emptying of tumor vessels
B. Stretching and deviation of vessels
C. Vessel size
D. Renal displacement
E. Portal vein involvement

Ref. Radiology 101:539, December, 1971

HEPATOMAS

759. WHICH OF THE FOLLOWING ARE USEFUL TESTS IN THE DIAGNOSIS OF PRIMARY HEPATOMAS IN CHILDREN?:
A. Alkaline phosphatase
B. Liver scan
C. Hypercholesterolemia
D. Alpha $_1$ fetoglobulin
E. Elevation of serum bilrubin

Ref. J Pediatr Surg 6:272, June, 1971

INTRACARDIAC TUMORS

760. THE PRESENCE OF CALCIFICATION WITHIN AN INTRACARDIAC TUMOR IN A INFANT AND CHILD LIMITS THE DIAGNOSIS TO WHICH OF THE FOLLOWING?:
A. Rhabdomyoma
B. Fibroma
C. Hemangioma
D. Teratoma
E. Myxoma

Ref. Br Heart J 33:125, January, 1971

NEUROBLASTOMA AND CEREBELLAR ENCEPHALOPATHY

761. IN ACUTE CEREBELLAR ENCEPHALOPATHY WHICH OF THE FOLLOWING DIAGNOSTIC AND LABORATORY PROCEDURES SHOULD BE DONE?:
A. Chest roentgenogram
B. Intravenous urogram
C. Skeletal survey
D. Bone marrow aspiration
E. Urinary catecholamines

Ref. J Pediatr 75:989, December, 1969

RETINOBLASTOMA

762. A NATIONWIDE STUDY OF 1623 HOSPITAL RECORDS OF CHILDREN WITH RETINOBLASTOMA REVEALED A SIGNIFICANT ASSOCIATION OF THIS TUMOR WITH WHICH OF THE FOLLOWING?:
A. Mental retardation
B. Major congenital malformations including the D-deletion syndrome
C. Secondary primary cancers
D. Bilateral involvement
E. Low incidence of inheritance from survivors of unilateral, sporadic retinoblastomas

Ref. N Engl J Med
285:307, August 5, 1971

RHABDOMYOSARCOMA

763. RHABDOMYOSARCOMA IS A HIGHLY MALIGNANT TUMOR IN THE PEDIATRIC AGE GROUP. ITS CLINICAL FEATURES AND FACTORS WHICH AFFECT LONG-TERM SURVIVAL INCLUDE WHICH OF THE FOLLOWING?:
A. Most common soft tissue sarcoma in infants and children
B. Most commonly seen in infants and preschool children
C. Worst survival rates in patients under one year
D. Best treatment regimen combines surgery, irradiation, and chemotherapy
E. Tumors that arise in orbit and extremities have higher survival rates

Ref. J Pediatr Surg
6:571, October, 1971

SACROCOCCYGEAL MASSES

764. THE PRESENCE OF A DIMPLE OR SINUS, HAIR CHANGES OR SKIN DISCOLORATION OVER A SKIN-COVERED SACROCOCCYGEAL MASS IN A NEWBORN SERVES TO DIFFERENTIATE WHICH OF THE FOLLOWING?:
A. Teratoma
B. Lipomeningocele
C. Lipoma
D. Meningocele
E. "Mixed neural" (myelocystoceles etc)

Ref. J Pediatr
79:948, December, 1971

765. ANTERIOR DISPLACEMENT OF THE RECTUM OF A NEWBORN INFANT MAY BE ASSOCIATED WITH WHICH OF THE FOLLOWING?:
A. Teratoma
B. Anterior meningocele
C. Neuroblastoma
D. Lipomeningocele
E. Lumbosacral lipoma

Ref. J Pediatr
79:948, December, 1971

766. PALPATION (CYSTIC, SOFT OR FIRM) AND THE SIZE OF SKIN-COVERED SACROCOCCYGEAL MASSES MAKE IT POSSIBLE TO CLINICALLY DIAGNOSE WHICH OF THE FOLLOWING?:
A. Teratoma
B. Lipomeningocele
C. Lipoma
D. Meningocele
E. "Mixed neural" (myelocystoceles etc)

Ref. J Pediatr
79:948, December, 1971

ONCOLOGIC SYNDROMES

ONCOLOGIC SYNDROMES ARE BEING IDENTIFIED WITH INCREASING FREQUENCY IN CHILDREN WITH A VARIETY OF CHROMOSOMAL, GENETIC AND CONSTITUTIONAL DISORDERS. MATCH THE NEOPLASTIC DISEASE WITH THE CLINICAL DIAGNOSIS:

A. Leukemia and lymphoma
B. Wilm's tumor
C. Carcinoma of the liver (hepatoblastoma or hepatoma)
D. Adrenal cortical carcinoma
E. Pheochromocytoma

767. ___ Beckwith's syndrome
768. ___ Ataxia-telangiectasia, hereditary
769. ___ Hemihypertrophy
770. ___ Down's syndrome
771. ___ Fanconi's syndrome (aplastic anemia with congenital anomalies)
772. ___ Bloom's syndrome
773. ___ Congenital sporadic aniridia
774. ___ Wiskott-Aldrich syndrome
775. ___ Von Hippel-Lindau
776. ___ Neurofibromatosis
777. ___ Chediak-Higashi syndrome
778. ___ D trisomy (13)

Ref. Natl Cancer Instit
32:221
Clin Pediatr
10:374, July, 1971

FOR EACH OF THE FOLLOWING MULTIPLE CHOICE QUESTIONS, SELECT THE ONE APPROPRIATE ANSWER:

ACCIDENTS IN TWINS

779. ACCIDENTS ARE THE LEADING CAUSE OF DEATH AMONG PRESCHOOL CHILDREN. IN A STUDY OF THE BEHAVIORAL ANTECEDENTS OF ACCIDENTAL INJURIES IN TWINS, ALL OF THE FOLLOWING WERE DEMONSTRATED, EXCEPT:

A. The number of accidents for boys equals the number of accidents for girls in preschoolers
B. After the age of three years there is a decline in the total number of accidents in children
C. The more temperamental and impulsive twin is more "accident-prone"
D. The amount of general activity is most strongly related to accident frequency
E. The less attentive and more easily distracted of the twins had more accidents

Ref. J Pediatr
79:122, July, 1971

BURNS

780. IN THE MANAGEMENT OF THE SEVERELY BURNED CHILD, ALL OF THE FOLLOWING APPEAR TO BE CORRECT, EXCEPT:

A. Mortality figures in the burned child have been favorably influenced by topical therapy
B. Heptavalent Pseudomonas vaccine appears to be a safe and effective agent in provoking significant antibody response
C. Antibody levels from active immunization to Pseudomonas diminish rapidly, presumably from loss of gamma globulin into the burn wound
D. Heptavalent-fortified globulin has shown promise in the passive immunization of the burned patient
E. The Pseudomonas vaccine does not affect the rate of skin colonization in burned children

Ref. J Pediatr Surg
6:547, October, 1971

CENTRAL VENOUS CATHETERS IN CHILDREN

781. USING A CENTRAL VENOUS CATHETER FOR MONITORING VENOUS PRESSURE OR FOR EXTENDED INTRAVENOUS FEEDING IS SAFE AND CAN BE LIFE PRESERVING. EACH OF THE FOLLOWING IS ACCEPTABLE WITH THE EXCEPTION OF:

A. A higher incidence of thrombo-embolism from the femoral vein and inferior vena cava makes this an undesirable site for a central venous line
B. A central venous pressure less than 5 cm of water indicates hypovolemia, which may result from actual blood or fluid loss or from "functional" loss such as intravascular pooling
C. A central venous pressure above 15 cm of water indicates hypervolemia from excessive blood or fluid administration, or congestive heart failure
D. Only radiopaque catheters should be used, and a chest X-ray should be taken immediately after placement to confirm that the catheter is in the right position
E. Percutaneous placement through a peripheral vein or via subclavian puncture is recommended as a safe procedure for all children including infants

Ref. Clin Pediatr
10:218, April, 1971

DERMATOGLYPHICS

782. APPROXIMATELY 2 PER CENT OF CHILDREN HAVE A SINGLE PALMAR CREASE. ALL OF THE FOLLOWING ARE CORRECT IN REGARD TO THE SPC, EXCEPT:

A. Children with an SPC have a significantly higher incidence of congenital abnormalities
B. Borderline or lower intellectual ability has a significant association with an SPC
C. There is a higher incidence of SPC among children with minimal cerebral dysfunction
D. Palmar crease abnormalities suggest an insult to the fetus in the first trimester
E. The recently described Sydney line has been found to have an association with childhood leukemia

Ref. Clin Pediatr
10:392, July, 1971

FEVER

783. MOST FEVERS IN CHILDREN ARE OF VIRAL ORIGIN, ARE SELF-LIMITED, AND ARE UNLIKELY TO BE ASSOCIATED WITH SERIOUS CONSEQUENCES. EACH OF THE FOLLOWING STATEMENTS CONCERNING FEVER IN CHILDREN IS CORRECT, EXCEPT:

A. Polymorphonuclear leukocytes release endogenous pyrogen in the inflammatory response which acts directly on the hypothalamic thermoregulatory center
B. No explanation exists for the febrile response of granulocytopenic patients
C. Many viruses stop multiplying in the temperature ranges which are induced by fever
D. Artificial elevation of the body temperature increases the survival rate in newborn dogs infected with canine herpesvirus
E. Most methods of external cooling of febrile children tend to increase oxygen demand and increase muscular activity through shivering

Ref. J Pediatr
77:935, November, 1970

FLUORESCENT STAINING OF HUMAN CHROMOSOMES

784. FLUORESCENT STAINING OF HUMAN CHROMOSOMES IS A MAJOR ADVANCE FOR CYTOGENETIC INVESTIGATORS. EACH OF THE FOLLOWING STATEMENTS IS CORRECT IN REGARD TO THIS NEW TECHNIQUE, EXCEPT:

A. The technique is not applicable to the study of the Y chromosome on a buccal smear
B. The Y chromosome appears to be the most brilliantly fluorescent of the chromosomes
C. It has now been demonstrated conclusively that the Philadelphia chromosome is No. 22
D. Bacteria which fluoresce may confuse the technique
E. The "extra" chromosome in Down's syndrome has now been identified as the G chromosome

Ref. Exp Cell Res
62:490, 1970
N Engl J Med
284:788

ELECTRICAL BURNS OF MOUTH

785. ELECTRICAL BURNS OF THE MOUTH CONSTITUTE A COMMON AND DESTRUCTIVE INJURY IN CHILDHOOD. EACH OF THE FOLLOWING IS CORRECT, EXCEPT:

A. Mouthing a live female extension cord plug is the most common mechanism of injury with the child's electrolyte rich saliva completing the electrical circuit
B. If the child's body is grounded (a wet diaper touching a radiator) cardiac arrest could occur
C. The extent of the electrical burn is apparent immediately and is associated with intense pain
D. Antibiotic usage has not influenced the incidence of infection and cellulitis
E. Children should be hospitalized for a full 21 days since serious and massive delayed bleeding may occur

Ref. Pediatrics
47:113, January, 1971

LYMPHANGIOGRAPHY

786. IN THE PAST FEW YEARS THE LIMITATIONS AND DANGERS OF LYMPHANGIOGRAPHY HAVE COME TO LIGHT. EACH OF THE FOLLOWING IS CORRECT, EXCEPT:

A. In abnormal lymph nodes lymphaticovenous communications may result in large amounts of contrast material getting into the lungs
B. The pulmonary complications of lymphangiography have included thromboembolic phenomena
C. A wide margin of safety exists in performing lymphangiography even in children with borderline pulmonary function
D. The usual X-ray finding after lymphangiographic examination is fine-granule stippling in both lungs
E. Chemical pneumonia occurs in a substantial number of patients after lymphangiography

Ref. N Engl J Med
284:899

READING DISORDERS

787. AN ESTIMATED 10 TO 20 PER CENT OF U.S. SCHOOL CHILDREN WITH NORMAL INTELLIGENCE SUFFER FROM READING PROBLEMS. EACH OF THE FOLLOWING IS CORRECT IN REGARD TO READING DISORDERS WHICH ARISE IN CHILDREN OF NORMAL INTELLIGENCE, EXCEPT:

A. Test data suggests that the tendency of prematurely born children to have difficulties in school may to some extent reflect the lack of stimulation which is imposed in most nurseries by current prolonged isolation practices
B. Little relationship exists between slow speech development and difficulty in learning to read and write
C. A thorough visual examination is critical for any child who is having difficulty learning to read
D. Boys suffer from reading disabilities far more commonly than girls
E. Among the most important factors which underlie reading problems of children with normal intelligence are: poor instruction, frequent changes of school, socioeconomic and environmental difficulties

Ref. Clin Pediatr
10:13A, April, 1971

RESTRAINT AND SPEECH

788. IN A STUDY OF CHILDREN WITH LANGUAGE AND SPEECH DISTURBANCES WHO HAD EXPERIENCED MOTOR RESTRAINT DURING EARLY LIFE, ALL OF THE FOLLOWING WERE DEMONSTRATED, EXCEPT:
A. No difference in the incidence of speech problems between males and females
B. No differences in children diagnosed as having neurological deficits from children with no evidence of central nervous system impairment
C. An increased incidence of speech problems in children with PKU with a history of physical immobilization over a matched group of children with PKU who had no history of physical restraint or sensory restriction
D. A direct relationship between the age of the initial restraint experience and the presence of language delay and articulation problems
E. No relationship between the duration of the initial restraint experience and the development of language problems

Ref. Pediatrics
48:116, July, 1971

SPEECH

789. THE MOST COMMON CAUSE OF DELAYED SPEECH IS:
A. Mental retardation
B. Childhood psychosis
C. Conduction deafness
D. Elective mutism
E. Aphasia

Ref. Pediatrics
47:327, 1971

SUDDEN DEATH SYNDROME

790. ATTEMPTS TO DEMONSTRATE EVIDENCE OF VIREMIA IN 119 UNSELECTED CASES OF THE SUDDEN DEATH SYNDROME OF INFANCY HAVE SHOWN WHICH OF THE FOLLOWING IN A SIGNIFICANT PERCENTAGE OF CASES?:
A. Influenza A_2
B. A variety of respiratory viruses including respiratory syncytial and herpes simplex
C. Enteroviruses including ECHO and Coxsackie B
D. No virus isolation but high levels of serum interferon
E. No virus isolation and rarely detectable levels of serum interferon

Ref. Pediatrics
48:79, July, 1971

SUICIDE

791. SUICIDE IS NOW THE THIRD LEADING CAUSE OF DEATH IN THE AGE GROUP 15-19 YEARS. IN A STUDY OF SELF-DESTRUCTIVE BEHAVIOUR IN CHILDREN ALL OF THE FOLLOWING WERE OBSERVED, EXCEPT:
A. After the age of 11 years, girls show an abrupt increase in self-poisoning
B. Self-poisoning before the age of 10 years is rarely intentional
C. Drug use for "kicks" or "trips" was rarely diagnosed as a suicide attempt
D. Toxicologic mishaps, rather than lethality of intent, are common
E. There is need for long-term follow-up of self-poisoning of children and adolescents

Ref. Clin Pediatr
10:414, July, 1971

FOR EACH OF THE FOLLOWING QUESTIONS, SELECT THE ONE APPROPRIATE ANSWER BY USING THE KEY OUTLINED BELOW:

1. If A, B and C are correct
2. If A and C are correct
3. If B and D are correct
4. If all are correct
5. If all are incorrect

ALPHA$_1$-FETOGLOBULIN

792. ALTHOUGH THERE MAY BE A RELATIVE QUANTITATIVE SPECIFICITY OF SERUM ALPHA$_1$-FETOGLOBULIN FOR PRIMARY HEPATOMAS, WHICH OF THE FOLLOWING TUMORS OR CLINICAL DISEASES HAVE HAD AN ASSOCIATION WITH THIS GLOBULIN?:
A. Systemic lupus erythematosus
B. Gastric adenocarcinoma
C. Granulomatous colitis
D. Embryonal testicular tumors
E. Wilms' tumor

Ref. N Engl J Med 285:1060, November 4, 1971

AMNIOCENTESIS

793. THE MAJORITY OF GENETIC SERVICES WOULD RECOMMEND AMNIOCENTESIS IN THE FOLLOWING CLINICAL SITUATIONS:
A. Family history of gene-transmitted or chromosomal abnormality
B. Parent with balanced chromosomal translocation
C. Advanced age of mother
D. Viral infection first trimester
E. History of exposure to mutagen(s)

Ref. Birth Defects National Foundation Page 49, September, 1971

FAT EMBOLISM

794. MASSIVE DOSES OF STEROIDS APPEAR TO BE EFFICACIOUS IN THE TREATMENT OF SEVERE FAT EMBOLISM. WHICH OF THE FOLLOWING SUGGEST THIS CLINICAL EMERGENCY?:
A. Lipuria
B. Hyperpyrexia
C. Pulmonary hypertension
D. Elevation of serum lipase
E. Petechiae

Ref. Surg Gynec Obstet 132:667, 1971

DROWNING

A NUMBER OF COMPLICATIONS MAY ARISE IN CHILDREN WHO HAVE SURVIVED NEAR-DROWNING, AND THE SEQUELAE RELATE TO WHETHER THE CHILD HAS ASPIRATED FRESH WATER OR SEA WATER.
MATCH THE FOLLOWING:
A. Fresh water
B. Sea water
C. Both
D. Neither

795. ___ Extensive hemolysis of erythrocytes
796. ___ Hypotension
797. ___ Acute tubular necrosis
798. ___ Hypertension
799. ___ Hemoconcentration
800. ___ Anoxia

Ref. JAMA 217:207, July 12, 1971

Some Questions and Answers on GARAMYCIN® Pediatric Injectable brand of gentamicin sulfate, U.S.P., injection 10 mg./cc.

Q. What are the current mortality rates in neonatal sepsis?

A. Mortality rates may be as high as 50 per cent with many commonly used antibiotics.[1-3]

Q. What is the most frequently encountered pathogen?

A. Studies indicate that over 40 per cent of neonatal infections are caused by *E. coli.*

Q. Is *E. coli* resistance rising?

A. Yes, a recent clinical study demonstrated the emergence of *E. coli* resistance to commonly used antibiotics in neonatal infections.

Please see pp. 191 and 192 for full prescribing information.

ANSWER KEY

The author has made every effort to thoroughly verify the questions and answers. However, in a volume of this size, some ambiguities and possible inaccuracies may appear. Therefore, if in doubt, consult your references.

THE PUBLISHERS

SECT. I

1. A
2. E
3. E
4. A
5. E
6. A
7. E
8. C
9. C
10. B
11. E
12. E
13. B
14. B
15. C
16. E
17. 1
18. 3
19. 5
20. 4
21. 4
22. 4
23. 4
24. 3
25. 1
26. 1
27. 1
28. 5
29. 1

SECT. II

30. C
31. A
32. A
33. C
34. B
35. A
36. C
37. A
38. C
39. C
40. C
41. F
42. D
43. E
44. I
45. H
46. J
47. A
48. B
49. G
50. A
51. C
52. C
53. B
54. B
55. A
56. C
57. C
58. B
59. B
60. B
61. A
62. C
63. B
64. A
65. B
66. A
67. C
68. E
69. E
70. E
71. A
72. A
73. A
74. A
75. E
76. C
77. E
78. C
79. A
80. A
81. B
82. C
83. B
84. E
85. D
86. 4
87. 4
88. 4
89. 2
90. 4
91. 4
92. 3
93. 1
94. 3
95. 4
96. 4
97. 4
98. 1
99. 4

Some Questions and Answers on GARAMYCIN® Pediatric Injectable brand of gentamicin sulfate, U.S.P., injection 10 mg./cc.

Q. **Has a similar pattern of *E. coli* resistance to gentamicin been demonstrated?**

A. No, because of its continuing efficacy against *E. coli* and most other susceptible gram-negative pathogens, GARAMYCIN Pediatric Injectable can be considered as initial therapy for suspected as well as documented gram-negative sepsis. In the neonate with suspected sepsis, a penicillin-type drug is usually indicated as concomitant antimicrobial therapy.

Q. **What is the antibacterial spectrum of GARAMYCIN Pediatric Injectable?**

A. GARAMYCIN Pediatric Injectable provides effective antibacterial activity against susceptible strains of the following microorganisms usually implicated in life-threatening infections: *Escherichia coli, Pseudomonas aeruginosa,* indole positive and negative *Proteus* species, *Klebsiella-Enterobacter-Serratia* species, and *Staphylococcus* species.

Please see pp. 191 and 192 for full prescribing information.

ANSWER KEY

100. 1
101. I
102. C
103. M
104. D
105. J
106. A
107. B
108. P
109. S
110. B
111. N
112. P
113. I
114. E
115. O
116. D
117. M
118. L
119. Q
120. F
121. A
122. N
123. K
124. C
125. V
126. P
127. S

SECT. III

128. C
129. B
130. B
131. C
132. A
133. C
134. C
135. E
136. A
137. D
138. B
139. D
140. C
141. A
142. E
143. B
144. B
145. E
146. D
147. A
148. C
149. E
150. D
151. C
152. B
153. A
154. D
155. B
156. C
157. E
158. D
159. C
160. E
161. D
162. 1
163. 2
164. 4

SECT. IV

165. A
166. E
167. E
168. A
169. D
170. E
171. A
172. A
173. E
174. E
175. C
176. D
177. A
178. A
179. E
180. A
181. E
182. A
183. E
184. B
185. B
186. C
187. A
188. E
189. E
190. C
191. A
192. D
193. E
194. A
195. B
196. B
197. C
198. D
199. 4
200. 4
201. 1

Some Questions and Answers on GARAMYCIN® Pediatric Injectable brand of gentamicin sulfate, U.S.P., injection 10 mg./cc.

Q. What are the indications for GARAMYCIN Pediatric Injectable?

A. GARAMYCIN Pediatric Injectable is recommended as initial therapy in suspected or documented gram-negative sepsis. Clinical studies have also shown the drug to be effective in septicemia and serious infections of the central nervous system (meningitis), urinary, respiratory and gastrointestinal tracts, skin and soft tissue (including burns), caused by sensitive pathogens.

In the neonate with suspected sepsis or staphylococcal pneumonia, a penicillin-type drug is usually indicated as concomitant antimicrobial therapy.

NOTE: The decision to continue GARAMYCIN therapy should be based on the results of susceptibility tests, the severity of infection and the important additional concepts in the "WARNING" box in the product information.

Please see pp. 191 and 192 for full prescribing information.

ANSWER KEY

202. 1
203. 4
204. 4
205. 1

SECT. V

206. C
207. E
208. B
209. D
210. C
211. E
212. D
213. E
214. B
215. C
216. A
217. A
218. C
219. C
220. A
221. D
222. B
223. E
224. C
225. B
226. C
227. A
228. B
229. A
230. B
231. A
232. 4
233. 2
234. 4
235. 4
236. 4
237. 1
238. 1
239. 1
240. 2
241. B
242. A
243. B
244. C
245. A
246. D
247. A
248. B
249. C
250. D
251. C
252. A
253. A
254. B
255. B
256. A

SECT. VI

257. A
258. A
259. A
260. A
261. E
262. D
263. A
264. A
265. D
266. D
267. A
268. E
269. C
270. B
271. E
272. C
273. E
274. D
275. E
276. A
277. B
278. D
279. 3
280. 1
281. 4
282. 4
283. 4
284. 4
285. 4
286. 4
287. 3
288. 4
289. 4
290. 1
291. 4
292. 4
293. 1
294. 1
295. D
296. C
297. B
298. A
299. E
300. C
301. A
302. D
303. C

Some Questions and Answers on GARAMYCIN® Pediatric Injectable brand of gentamicin sulfate, U.S.P., injection 10 mg./cc.

Q. **Can GARAMYCIN Pediatric Injectable be used in gram-positive or mixed infections?**

A. Yes. GARAMYCIN Pediatric Injectable has been shown to be effective in serious staphylococcal infections. The drug may be considered in these cases when the organism is resistant to the penicillins, or when other less potentially toxic drugs are contraindicated. It may also be considered in mixed infections caused by susceptible strains of *Staphylococcus aureus* and gram-negative organisms.

Please see pp. 191 and 192 for full prescribing information.

ANSWER KEY

304. B
305. A

SECT. VII

306. E
307. C
308. B
309. D
310. C
311. E
312. E
313. A
314. A
315. D
316. D
317. E
318. A
319. D
320. D
321. D
322. D
323. E
324. 4
325. 3
326. 4
327. D
328. C
329. A
330. C
331. A
332. A
333. C
334. C
335. A
336. C
337. A
338. B
339. B,D
340. E
341. C
342. C
343. A
344. A,D
345. A,E
346. B,F
347. E
348. F

SECT. VIII

349. A
350. C
351. E
352. D
353. A
354. A
355. D
356. D
357. A
358. E
359. D
360. A
361. E
362. D
363. C
364. A
365. B
366. E
367. D
368. A
369. C
370. D
371. E
372. A
373. D
374. D
375. B
376. C
377. C
378. B
379. E
380. E
381. B
382. E
383. C
384. E
385. E
386. D
387. D
388. C
389. B
390. A
391. B
392. A
393. D
394. E
395. D
396. A
397. D
398. A
399. A
400. B
401. D
402. C
403. D
404. 1
405. 1

Some Questions and Answers on GARAMYCIN® Pediatric Injectable brand of gentamicin sulfate, U.S.P., injection 10 mg./cc.

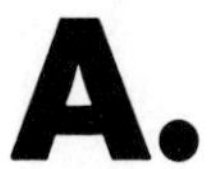

How rapidly are peak serum levels achieved?

A.

GARAMYCIN Pediatric Injectable, administered intramuscularly, provides prompt antibacterial activity. Peak serum concentrations occur generally between 30 to 90 minutes. In infants with normal renal function a single dose of 2.5 mg./kg. usually produces peak serum levels ranging from 3 to 5 mcg./ml. Measurable GARAMYCIN activity persists in serum for 8 to 12 hours.

When administered by intravenous infusion over a two-hour period, the peak serum concentration is similar to that resulting from the same dose given intramuscularly.

Please see pp. 191 and 192 for full prescribing information.

ANSWER KEY

406. 4
407. 4
408. 4
409. 1
410. 5
411. 4
412. 4
413. 4
414. 4
415. 5
416. 4
417. 4
418. 3
419. 5
420. 3
421. 4
422. 4
423. 4
424. 1
425. 4
426. 3
427. 3
428. 4
429. D
430. A
431. E
432. B
433. B
434. E
435. D
436. C
437. A
438. A
439. A
440. B
441. C
442. E
443. A
444. B
445. D
446. E
447. E
448. A
449. B
450. A
451. C
452. B
453. C
454. A
455. A
456. B
457. A
458. C
459. C
460. C
461. B
462. C
463. C
464. B
465. C
466. B

SECT. IX

467. E
468. A
469. E
470. A
471. D
472. E
473. B
474. C
475. A
476. A
477. A
478. E
479. C
480. D
481. B
482. D
483. C
484. E
485. 4
486. 4
487. 3
488. 4
489. 1
490. 4
491. 2
492. 5
493. 4
494. 1
495. B
496. A
497. A
498. B
499. A
500. A
501. B
502. B
503. A
504. A

SECT. X

505. C
506. B
507. E

Some Questions and Answers on GARAMYCIN® Pediatric Injectable brand of gentamicin sulfate, U.S.P., injection 10 mg./cc.

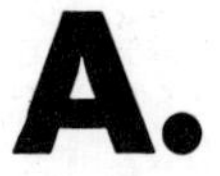

What are the recommended dosage guidelines for GARAMYCIN Pediatric Injectable?

A.

GARAMYCIN Pediatric Injectable may be administered either I.M. or I.V. The dosage guidelines in patients with normal renal function are identical for both routes of administration.

Infants and Neonates*

Total daily dose: 6 mg./kg./day administered in two equal doses every 12 hours, or three equal doses every 8 hours.

**NOTE: Premature or Full Term Neonates One Week of Age or Less: the total daily dose should be administered in two equal doses every 12 hours.*

Children

3 to 5 mg./kg./day divided into three equal doses every 8 hours.

Please see pp. 191 and 192 for full prescribing information.

ANSWER KEY

508. C
509. D
510. D
511. B
512. D
513. C
514. C
515. C
516. B
517. B
518. A
519. D
520. C
521. A
522. C
523. E
524. D
525. B
526. B
527. E
528. E
529. B
530. D
531. D
532. E
533. B
534. E
535. A
536. D
537. A
538. 1
539. 1
540. 4
541. 2
542. 4
543. 4
544. 3
545. 4
546. 2
547. 4
548. 2
549. 4
550. D
551. B
552. A
553. A
554. B
555. A
556. C
557. A
558. A
559. A
560. C
561. B
562. A
563. A
564. A
565. B
566. A
567. B
568. C
569. A
570. C
571. A
572. B
573. B
574. D
575. A
576. E
577. C

SECT. XI

578. E
579. B
580. B
581. D
582. E
583. B
584. A
585. E
586. B
587. 4
588. 2
589. 3
590. 2
591. 4
592. D
593. H
594. B
595. C
596. A
597. G
598. F
599. E

SECT. XII

600. E
601. B
602. C
603. A
604. A
605. D
606. A
607. D
608. A
609. D

Some Questions and Answers on GARAMYCIN® Pediatric Injectable brand of gentamicin sulfate, U.S.P., injection 10 mg./cc.

Q. What is the usual duration of therapy?

A. The usual duration of treatment is 7 to 10 days. In difficult and complicated infections, a longer course of therapy may be necessary. In such cases monitoring of renal function and of auditory and vestibular functions when feasible is advisable, since neurotoxicity is more apt to occur with prolonged treatment.

Q. Does GARAMYCIN Pediatric Injectable have a cumulative effect?

A. No. GARAMYCIN Pediatric Injectable does not accumulate in the serum of patients with normal renal function. In patients with impaired or immature renal function, however, the serum half-life is prolonged and dosage must be adjusted accordingly.

Please see pp. 191 and 192 for full prescribing information.

ANSWER KEY

610. E
611. C
612. A
613. 5
614. 5
615. B
616. C
617. D
618. F
619. E
620. A
621. B
622. A
623. D
624. C
625. A

SECT. XIII

626. E
627. D
628. A
629. E
630. D
631. E
632. B
633. A
634. B
635. A
636. C
637. B
638. E
639. A
640. B
641. A
642. A
643. C
644. B
645. D
646. D
647. C
648. D
649. A
650. E
651. A
652. D
653. 1
654. 4
655. 1
656. 2
657. 4
658. 1
659. 4
660. 4
661. 4
662. 4
663. 4
664. 4
665. C
666. A
667. C
668. A
669. B

SECT. XIV

670. A
671. B
672. A
673. D
674. E
675. E
676. B
677. 1
678. 4
679. 1
680. 4
681. 4
682. 4

SECT. XV

683. E
684. D
685. D
686. D
687. A
688. E
689. B
690. B
691. A
692. D
693. D
694. B
695. A
696. E
697. A
698. E
699. E
700. A
701. B
702. D
703. A
704. C
705. B
706. D
707. E

Some Questions and Answers on GARAMYCIN® Pediatric Injectable brand of gentamicin sulfate, U.S.P., injection 10 mg./cc.

Q. **Are there guidelines for adjusting the dosage of GARAMYCIN Pediatric Injectable in patients with impaired renal function?**

A. Yes. The single dose of GARAMYCIN Pediatric Injectable given by patient weight remains the same; however, the interval between doses must be extended.

This interval may be approximated by multiplying the serum creatinine by eight as follows:

Serum Creatinine x 8 = frequency of administration
(mg./100 ml.) (in hours)

This dosage schedule is not intended as a rigid recommendation, but is provided as a guide to dosage when the measurement of gentamicin serum levels is not feasible.

Q. **Can bacterial resistance to GARAMYCIN Pediatric Injectable be expected to develop rapidly?**

A. No. Bacterial resistance to GARAMYCIN Pediatric Injectable has not been a problem. No one-step mutations to high resistance have been reported to date. However, slow stepwise resistance has developed in the laboratory when microorganisms are serially subcultured with the drug.

Please see pp. 191 and 192 for full prescribing information.

ANSWER KEY

708. C
709. A
710. A
711. A
712. D
713. B
714. E
715. C
716. B
717. D
718. E
719. B
720. A
721. D
722. 4
723. 3
724. 4
725. 4
726. 1
727. 3
728. 4
729. 4
730. 4
731. 1
732. 4
733. 1
734. 1
735. D
736. B
737. A
738. D
739. B
740. A
741. F
742. C
743. H
744. D
745. E
746. G

SECT. XVI

747. E
748. E
749. E
750. D
751. B
752. A
753. A
754. E
755. E
756. A
757. B
758. 5
759. 3
760. 3
761. 4
762. 4
763. 4
764. 5
765. 1
766. 5
767. B,C,D
768. A
769. B,C,D
770. A
771. A
772. A
773. B
774. A
775. E
776. E
777. A
778. A

SECT. XVII

779. A
780. A
781. E
782. C
783. B
784. A
785. C
786. C
787. B
788. B
789. A
790. E
791. B
792. 3
793. 1
794. 4
795. A
796. C
797. C
798. D
799. B
800. C

Some Questions and Answers on GARAMYCIN® Pediatric Injectable brand of gentamicin sulfate, U.S.P., injection 10 mg./cc.

Q.

What about adverse reactions to GARAMYCIN Pediatric Injectable?

A.

GARAMYCIN Pediatric Injectable seems to be well tolerated in neonates, infants and children. The risk of toxic reactions is low, especially in patients with normal renal function who do not receive the drug at higher doses or for longer than recommended periods of time.

See "WARNING" box for statement on ototoxicity and nephrotoxicity

References

1. *Finland, M.: Discussion, J. Infect. Dis. 124 (suppl.): S 260, 1971.*
2. *Klein, J.O.: Consideration of gentamicin for therapy of neonatal sepsis, J. Infect. Dis. 119:457, 1969.*
3. *Klein, J.O.; Herschel, M.; Therakan, R.M., and Ingall, D.: Gentamicin in serious neonatal infections: Absorption, excretion and clinical results in 25 cases, J. Infect. Dis. 124 (suppl.): S 224, 1971.*

Please see pp. 191 and 192 for full prescribing information.

Other Products from Schering:

DEMAZIN® REPETABS® Tablets
brand of chlorpheniramine maleate,
U.S.P. and phenylephrine

DEMAZIN® Syrup
brand of chlorpheniramine maleate,
U.S.P. and phenylephrine hydrochloride, U.S.P.

A and D Cream
REG. T.M.

A and D Ointment
REG. T.M.

VALISONE® Cream
brand of betamethasone valerate, N.F.

VALISONE® Ointment
brand of betamethasone valerate, N.F.

VALISONE® Aerosol
brand of betamethasone valerate, N.F.

Garamycin® Pediatric Injectable
brand of gentamicin sulfate, U.S.P., Injection
10 mg per cc
Each cc contains gentamicin sulfate equivalent to 10 mg gentamicin
For Parenteral Administration

WARNING

Patients treated with GARAMYCIN Pediatric Injectable should be under close clinical observation because of the potential toxicity associated with the use of this drug.

Ototoxicity, both vestibular and auditory, can occur in patients, primarily those with pre-existing renal damage, treated with GARAMYCIN Pediatric Injectable usually for longer periods or with higher doses than recommended.

GARAMYCIN Pediatric Injectable is potentially nephrotoxic, and this should be kept in mind particularly when it is used in patients with pre-existing renal impairment.

Monitoring of renal and eighth nerve function is recommended during therapy of patients with known impairment of renal function. This testing is also recommended in patients with normal renal function at onset of therapy who develop evidence of nitrogen retention (increasing BUN, NPN, creatinine or oliguria). Evidence of ototoxicity requires dosage adjustments or discontinuance of the drug.

In event of overdose or toxic reactions, peritoneal dialysis or hemodialysis will aid in removal of gentamicin from the blood. In the newborn infant exchange transfusions may also be considered.

Serum concentrations should be monitored when feasible and prolonged concentrations above 12 mcg/ml should be avoided.

Concurrent use of other neurotoxic and/or nephrotoxic drugs, particularly streptomycin, neomycin, kanamycin, cephaloridine, viomycin, polymixin B, and polymyxin E (colistin), should be avoided.

The concurrent use of gentamicin with potent diuretics should be avoided, since certain diuretics by themselves may cause ototoxicity. In addition, when administered intravenously, diuretics may cause a rise in gentamicin serum level and potentiate neurotoxicity.

DESCRIPTION Gentamicin sulfate, U.S.P., a water soluble antibiotic of the aminoglycoside group, is derived from a strain of *Micromonospora purpurea,* an actinomycete. GARAMYCIN Pediatric Injectable is a sterile aqueous solution containing in each cc gentamicin sulfate equivalent to 10 mg gentamicin base, 1.3 mg methylparaben, U.S.P., and 0.2 mg propylparaben, U.S.P., as preservatives, 3.2 mg sodium bisulfite, U.S.P., and 0.1 mg disodium edetate, U.S.P. GARAMYCIN Pediatric Injectable is stable and requires no refrigeration.

ACTIONS After intramuscular administration of GARAMYCIN Pediatric Injectable, peak serum concentrations usually occur between 30 and 90 minutes. In infants a single dose of 2.5 mg/kg usually provides a peak serum level in the range of 3 to 5 mcg/ml. Measurable gentamicin activity persists in serum for 8 to 12 hours.

In infants one week to 6 months of age, the half-life is 3 to 3½ hours. In full term and large premature infants less than one week old, the approximate serum half-life of gentamicin is 5½ hours. In small premature infants, the half-life is inversely related to birth weight. In premature infants weighing less than 1500 grams, the half-life is 11½ hours; in those weighing 1500 to 2000 grams, the half-life is 8 hours; in those weighing over 2000 grams, the half-life is approximately 5 hours.

Gentamicin administered every 8 to 12 hours does not accumulate in the serum of patients with normal renal function. In patients with impaired or immature renal function, the serum half-life is prolonged, and dosage must be adjusted. When gentamicin is administered by intravenous infusion over a 2-hour period, the peak serum concentration is similar to that resulting from the same dose administered intramuscularly. The serum half-life of gentamicin following intravenous infusion is shorter than after intramuscular administration.

Approximately 25 to 30% of the administered dose of gentamicin is bound by serum protein; it is released as the drug is excreted. Gentamicin is excreted principally by glomerular filtration in the urine. Consequently, urine concentrations are high. In neonates less than 3 days old, approximately 10% of the administered dose is excreted in 12 hours; in infants 5 to 40 days old, approximately 40% is excreted over the same period. Excretion of gentamicin correlates with postnatal age and creatinine clearance. Thus, with increasing postnatal age and concomitant increase in renal maturity, gentamicin is excreted more rapidly.

Following parenteral administration, gentamicin can be detected in tissues and body fluids. Gentamicin crosses the peritoneal as well as the placental membranes. Concentrations in bile, in general, have been low which suggests minimal biliary excretion.

Gentamicin has also been found in the cerebrospinal fluid in minimal amounts. It has been found in sputum, pleural fluid, and peritoneal fluid.

INDICATIONS GARAMYCIN Pediatric Injectable is indicated with due regard for relative toxicity of antibiotics, in the treatment of serious infections caused by susceptible strains of the following microorganisms: *Pseudomonas aeruginosa, Proteus* species (indole positive and indole negative), *Escherichia coli, Klebsiella-Enterobacter-Serratia* species, and *Staphylococcus* species.

Clinical studies have shown GARAMYCIN Pediatric Injectable to be effective in septicemia and serious infections of the central nervous system (meningitis), urinary tract, respiratory tract, gastrointestinal tract, skin, and soft tissue (including burns).

In suspected or documented gram-negative sepsis, GARAMYCIN Pediatric Injectable may be considered as initial therapy. The decision to continue therapy with this drug should be based on the results of susceptibility tests, the severity of the infection, and the important additional concepts contained in the "Warning Box" on page one. In the neonate with suspected sepsis or staphylococcal pneumonia, a penicillin type drug is usually indicated as concomitant antimicrobial therapy.

GARAMYCIN Pediatric Injectable has been shown to be effective in serious staphylococcal infections. It may be considered in those infections when the organism is resistant to the penicillins or when other less potentially toxic drugs are contraindicated. It may also be considered in mixed infections caused by susceptible strains of *Staphylococcus aureus* and gram-negative organisms.

Bacteriologic tests to determine the causative organisms and their susceptibility to gentamicin should be performed.

Bacterial resistance to gentamicin develops slowly in stepwise fashion; there have been no one-step mutations to high resistance.

CONTRAINDICATIONS A history of hypersensitivity to gentamicin is a contraindication to its use.

WARNINGS (See WARNING BOX above.)

PRECAUTIONS Neuromuscular blockade and respiratory paralysis may occur with gentamicin especially if it is administered to patients receiving neuromuscular blocking agents such as succinylcholine or tubocurarine. Calcium or neostigmine may reverse these phenomena.

Treatment with gentamicin may result in overgrowth of nonsusceptible organisms. If this occurs, appropriate therapy is indicated.

ADVERSE REACTIONS

Nephrotoxicity: Adverse renal effects, as demonstrated by rising BUN, NPN, serum creatinine, and oliguria, have been reported. They occur more frequently in patients with a history of renal impairment usually treated with larger than recommended dosage.

Neurotoxicity: Adverse effects on both vestibular and auditory branches of the eighth nerve have been reported usually in patients on high dosage and/or prolonged therapy. Symptoms include dizziness, vertigo, tinnitus, roaring in the ears, and more rarely hearing loss.

Numbness, skin tingling, muscle twitching, and convulsions have also been reported.

Note: Gentamicin appears to be well tolerated in neonates, infants, and children. The risk of toxic reactions is low especially in patients with normal renal function who do not receive the drug at higher doses or for longer periods of time than recommended.

Other reported adverse reactions, possibly related to gentamicin, include increased serum transaminase (SGOT, SGPT), increased serum bilirubin, transient hepatomegaly, decreased serum calcium; splenomegaly, anemia, increased and decreased reticulocyte counts, granulocytopenia, thrombocytopenia, purpura; fever, rash, itching, urticaria, generalized burning, joint pain, laryngeal edema; nausea, vomiting, headache, increased salivation, lethargy and decreased appetite, weight loss, pulmonary fibrosis, hypotension, and hypertension.

DOSAGE AND ADMINISTRATION GARAMYCIN Pediatric Injectable may be given intramuscularly or intravenously.

For Intramuscular Administration:

PATIENTS WITH NORMAL RENAL FUNCTION

Children: 3 to 5 mg/kg/day administered in three equal doses every 8 hours.

Infants and Neonates: 6 mg/kg/day administered as two equal doses every 12 hours, or 3 equal doses every 8 hours.

Premature or Full Term Neonates One Week of Age or Less: The total daily dose should be administered in two equal doses every 12 hours.

The usual duration of treatment is 7 to 10 days. In difficult and complicated infections, a longer course of therapy may be necessary. In such cases monitoring of renal function and of auditory and vestibular functions when feasible is advisable, since neurotoxicity is more apt to occur with treatment extended over 10 days.

PATIENTS WITH IMPAIRED RENAL FUNCTION

Dosage must be adjusted in patients with impaired renal function. Since the creatinine clearance rate and serum creatinine concentration have high correlation with the serum half-life of gentamicin, these laboratory tests may provide the guidance necessary for adjustments of gentamicin dosage. In adults the serum half-life (in hours) of gentamicin may be estimated by multiplying the serum creatinine (mg %) by four. The frequency of administration (in hours) may be approximated by doubling the serum half-life or by multiplying the serum creatinine by eight. These guidelines may be considered when treating infants and children with serious renal impairment.

When GARAMYCIN Pediatric Injectable is indicated in children with renal failure undergoing 14-hour hemodialysis twice weekly, the recommended dosage is 2 mg/kg at the end of each dialysis period.

These guidelines are not intended as rigid recommendations, but are presented as an aid to dosage when the measurement of gentamicin serum levels is not feasible. They should be used in conjunction with close clinical and laboratory monitoring of the patient and modified as deemed necessary by the treating physician.

For Intravenous Administration:

The intravenous administration of GARAMYCIN Pediatric Injectable is recommended in those circumstances when the intramuscular route is not feasible (e.g., patients in shock, with hematologic disorders, with severe burns, or with markedly reduced muscle mass).

For intravenous administration a single dose of GARAMYCIN Pediatric Injectable may be diluted in sterile isotonic saline solution or in a sterile solution of dextrose 5% in water. The concentration of gentamicin in solution should normally not exceed 1 mg/cc (0.1%). The solution is infused over a period of 1 to 2 hours.

The recommended dose for intravenous administration is identical to that recommended for intramuscular use.

GARAMYCIN Pediatric Injectable should not be physically premixed with other drugs but should be administered separately in accordance with the recommended route of administration and dosage schedule.

HOW SUPPLIED GARAMYCIN Pediatric Injectable, 10 mg per cc, 2 cc multiple-dose vials, for parenteral administration.

Also available, Garamycin Injectable, 40 mg/cc, 2 cc multiple-dose vials, for parenteral administration.

MARCH, 1972

GA 337-11.72

Schering Corporation
Bloomfield, N.J. 07003